RELIEF FROM ARTHRITIS

This book is about the oceans and the treatment of arthritis, and in particular a new treatment from an extract taken from the New Zealand Green-Lipped Mussel which has proved effective in relieving the symptoms of arthritis.

RELIEF FROM ARTHRITIS
The Natural Way

by

JOHN E. CROFT
L.R.C.S., F.R.S.H.

THORSONS PUBLISHING GROUP
Wellingborough, Northamptonshire

Rochester, Vermont

First published 1979
Fifth impression 1984
Second edition, completely revised and reset, October 1986

British Library Cataloguing in Publication Data

Croft, John E.
  Relief from arthritis: the natural way.
  1. Arthritis — Treatment
  I. Title
  616.7'2206   RC933

ISBN 0-7225-1377-1

Printed and bound in Great Britain

Contents

Foreword

In future years when treatments from the sea are effectively combating many of our most serious and debilitating diseases, it will be interesting to recall that one of the first of these treatments was the New Zealand green mussel extract.

It is not unreasonable to expect that remedies for such disorders as multiple sclerosis, acquired immune deficiency syndrome and cancer will be discovered in the sea. Those who would challenge this statement need only consider that some eighty per cent of the biological productivity of the world, involving a greater diversity of life forms than on land, occurs in the seas.

Accepting the fact that many of our present medications originated in the jungles of the world it is easy to see, taking into account the point made in the previous paragraph, that the seas and oceans have, potentially, so much more to offer. It is interesting to note from the medicinal point of view that therapeutic substances derived from marine plants or animals are often highly potent and highly selective in their medicinal properties. This can be a very valuable asset in the treatment of clinical disorders.

This book results from thirteen years research and experience with the New Zealand mussel extract product. From its introduction to arthritis sufferers in New Zealand in the early seventies with much scepticism and opposition amongst the medical profession, the product has, as a result of its own success, now reached the stage where it is distributed across the world, is used by, and receives considerable support from, the medical profession and has even received Government funding for further research.

   In a period when some drug therapies for arthritis that were fully approved have had to be removed from sale because they have side effects that result in the death of patients, it should be a source of encouragement to sufferers of arthritis to know that safe and effective treatments, such as the one described in this book, are available and worth trying.

J. E. Croft
Auckland, New Zealand
March, 1986.

Introduction

There is nothing particularly new about the use of preparations made from the sea or its contents in medicine. For centuries crude extracts of marine plants and animals have been used to treat disease.

It was not until the 1960s however, long after space exploration began, that serious exploration of the marine environment for substances exhibiting pharmacologically active properties was undertaken. As a result of some of this work, the anti-inflammatory properties of a preparation extracted from the New Zealand green mussel were discovered. The work that followed the discovery and the subsequent success of the product, which was first distributed for general public use in New Zealand in 1974, forms the basis of this book.

One of the most influential factors in determining the genuine value of natural substances or preparations used for medicinal purposes is the use of these by ancient civilizations or so-called 'primitive' tribal groups still isolated from modern society. This is because the substances or preparations were, and in some cases still are, used almost entirely on the basis of experience.

There is no question of financial gain, scientific prestige, political or commercial pressure. Therefore, the only possible reason for the use of such preparations is that they were effective. Unfortunately this cannot be said of some of the modern, synthetic preparations in use today.

Many of the original tribal medicines have been fully investigated to reveal the biologically active molecule responsible for the medicinal value. This has then been followed by synthesization of the 'active' molecule for use in modern medicine. Some natural medicines however have defied scientific efforts to reproduce their activity synthetically. In certain cases this has been due to the fact that the molecular structure involved has been too complex to synthesize economically. In other cases the 'active' molecule has simply been too unstable when isolated from the parent substance. This is the situation with the New Zealand green mussel extract and is the reason for its continued preparation as a relatively crude extract even after such a long period of investigation.

Whenever a successful product is developed, imitation products follow closely behind. However, the mussel extract product, the only one to which the research and information in this book applies, is produced to a patented method and can be distinguished from imitations quite readily by a laboratory assay technique.

This book is based on information gathered over thirteen years, some of the information resulting from scientific and clinical research carried out in centres from Paris to Melbourne, and some from the direct communications of people in countries all around the world who have experienced the beneficial effects of the mussel extract.

Finally it might be asked why a book about an extract from a New Zealand shellfish need be written at all? Two reasons are put forward to answer such a question.

Firstly, this product could represent the first time in history that the sea has been actively farmed to produce a substance that is used to treat such a widespread and serious disease. This operation involves the application and monitoring of natural biological cycles in marine cultivation, water pollution control, factory processing and both clinical and laboratory research. The second reason relates to the fact that the author has so often been asked to talk on the subject with the almost inevitable response being, 'What a fascinating story, why don't you write a book about it?' The tale, then, is worthy of the telling.

Note:
The author wishes it to be understood that the information in this book relates only to the New Zealand mussel extract which has been the subject of all the published research. No responsibility is accepted for any imitation products which may be claimed to be the same material.

1
The Sea

In this chapter the nature and composition of the sea and some aspects of its use and value as a source of medication and healing are discussed.

As the seas cover some three-quarters of the surface of our planet, support a much greater quantity and variety of biological life forms than does the land mass, control the environmental conditions such that human life may exist and are quite capable of independently supporting human life, it is not unreasonable to believe that they may also provide a valuable source of medicinal substances.

In fact this belief is soundly based because the seas contain all the forms and combinations of elements and compounds needed for the treatment of disease. Some of the therapeutic properties of the seas have been known and used since biblical times and are still in use today. There are others, however, still to be discovered, and some which we know but cannot yet isolate and identify.

The statistically minded may be interested to know that the depth of the seas is so great that the total amount of land occupying the earth's surface could be submerged without even the highest mountains showing. The volume of water has been estimated to be of the order of 300 million cubic miles, with a weight of about 1,500 million, billion tons, or 1,524 million, billion tonnes!

The productivity of the seas in terms of biological life is much greater than that of the land. This may seem hard to believe if we think of the productivity of the tropical rain forests of the Amazon Basin or the African jungle. However, when put into perspective it is easy to understand. The jungles and rain forests occupy only small areas of the land surface, much of it being covered by desert, mountains and the concrete and brick of civilization. In fact about 80 per cent of the biological productivity on earth occurs in the sea.

Not only is the amount of living matter so much greater in the sea but also the variety of life forms, both plant and animal, is greater than it is on shore. A simple way to gain at least a little appreciation of these factors is to view a few small drops of sea water under a microscope at about 50 times magnification. A range of life forms, some resembling miniature dinosaurs, others looking like beautifully symmetrical, three-dimensional artistic works, will be seen. These

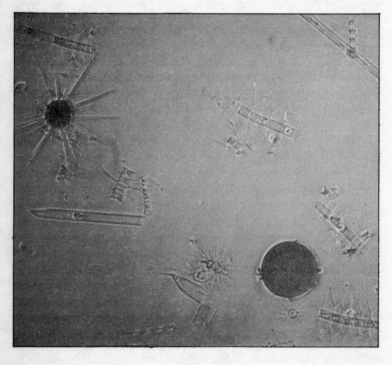

Figure 1.   Microscopic view of plankton

will be just a minute sample of the animals and plants forming the microscopic fraction of the marine plankton.

Another interesting feature of the productive activity of the sea is that by far the greatest production occurs in the shallow coastal waters. This is because the environment in these regions is suitable for more species to inhabit and the nutritional value of the waters is generally higher than in the deep oceans. The geographical distribution of life in the sea differs between tropical and colder waters. In the tropical regions there is a great diversity of species though not in particularly high populations whilst the colder waters support very large populations but with much less variety of species present.

Because they are of such immense volume and spread so widely over the earth's surface the seas have a very significant regulating influence on our atmospheric conditions. It is true to say that human life would not be able to exist on earth if it were not for the moderating influence of the oceans on surface temperatures. In addition the interchange of gases such as oxygen and carbon dioxide between the seas and the atmosphere is an important factor in maintaining the global balance of the atmosphere necessary to support both plant and animal life.

Additionally, most of the waste products of animal (this includes human) life eventually finish up in the sea, where, in general, they are rendered innocuous or are utilized. This is a general statement and certainly does not apply to all the wastes produced by the activities of the human animal. The subject of pollution of the seas is addressed in more detail later in this chapter, and in Chapter 6.

It has already been said that the sea can support human life. This is perfectly true and has been proven several times by the survival of shipwreck victims for many weeks without food or water stores. By drinking the freshwater content of the eyes of sea creatures such as turtles, or crudely distilling fresh water from salt water, using the sun's heat, human body fluids have been maintained. The flesh of fish and the cells of algae have provided sufficient nutrition to maintain life. This is not to imply that living from the sea alone is desirable; it is not, but it will at least sustain human life.

The Composition of the Seas

Away from the immediate influence of land or ice the seas have a reasonably uniform and consistent composition. Naturally there are local influences in some regions which significantly change the composition of the sea water. One example of this would be in the South Atlantic Ocean, off the north-east coast of Brazil, where the influence of the freshwater flow from the Amazon River is detectable up to 200 miles out to sea. Another example of freshwater dilution occurs in the vicinity of large masses of melting ice. These types of influences lead to stratification of the water column, with the water becoming saltier as the depth increases. Quite the reverse situation can occur in some equatorial regions where evaporation at the sea surface causes the salt content to increase.

The movement of the earth, winds and currents can also influence the composition of the sea water in some regions by creating upwellings, stratification layers, pronounced drift of water masses and so on.

In the main body of oceanic waters, however, the major constituents would be found in the amounts shown in Table 1. Some of the elements are present in amounts adequate for commercial extraction processes to operate. One such element for which shore-based commercial extraction takes place is bromine. The bromine extracted from the sea is usually used in the production of ethylene bromide for use as an additive in petroleum products.

There is also an enormous quantity of gold in the seas, (apart from that sitting in the vaults of the *Titanic* and a few Spanish galleons), but the volume of water to be processed in order to recover it would make any extraction process uneconomical.

| Chloride | 19,000 | Rubidium | 0.2 |
| Sodium | 10,500 | Lithium | 0.1 |

Magnesium	1,300	Phosphorus	0.1
Sulphur	900	Barium	0.05
Calcium	400	Iodide	0.05
Potassium	380	Arsenic	0.02
Bromide	65	Iron	0.02
Carbon	28	Copper	0.005
Strontium	13	Zinc	0.005
Boron	4.5	Lead	0.004
Silicon	4.0	Uranium	0.003
Fluoride	1.4	Vanadium	0.0003
Aluminium	0.5	Gold	0.000001

Table 1. Some of the constituents of sea water in order of approximate concentration present expressed in parts per million. N. B. Geographical situations cause variations in the above figures.

The Sea in Nutrition and as a Healer

The subject of the therapeutic properties of the sea and its flora and fauna is too extensive to cover adequately in a little book such as this. However, a few examples of these properties will demonstrate the sea's tremendous therapeutic potential.

It was a common practice of seamen in early times to drink small quantities of sea water to treat stomach disorders. They would apparently take up to half a small cupful of clean sea water regularly for several days to effect a satisfactory treatment. It was also a normal practice for wounds, scalds or burns to be immersed in clean sea water for both an antibiotic and rapid healing effect. This practice still goes on today. In fact some recent publicity has been given to the outstanding work of Sir Archibald McIndoe the famous plastic surgeon who successfully treated so many of the World War Two burn victims. Part of Sir Archibald's treatment involved the soaking of his badly burned patients in a saltwater bath not only to ease the removal of bandages, but to effect relief from pain plus better healing results than would otherwise be the case. The idea for this system of treatment came about through the observation that badly burned aircraftsmen who had baled out from their plane and landed in the sea showed better healing results than their colleagues who landed on shore.

Anyone who has received an abrasion or cut when swimming in the sea should have noticed that the affliction heals cleanly and quickly without need for medication. This is due to the excellent antibiotic properties of sea water. Seawater baths have also been claimed to help patients suffering from some forms of psoriasis.

It is notable too that animals and poultry which have access to the sea-shore and coastal fields to graze or feed are found to yield better meat and richer-yolked eggs.

Some commercial animals such as racehorses are nowadays regularly taken to swim in mineral baths as part of their training and health enhancement programme. The ideal mineral bath is of course the sea, but where access to the sea is not practicable, salts are added to the special pools designed for these animals to swim in. It is fair to comment that, whilst the addition of salts to these freshwater pools is advantageous it cannot compete for value with the natural mineral balance of sea water.

The same may be said of the spa pools in which people immerse themselves for the relief of some disorders. Most spas will have an excess of some mineral elements and a deficiency of others. In comparison seawater immersion provides all the mineral elements, all in solution, no excesses.

In regions of the Pacific and the West Indies, although the practice was probably not limited to these regions, it was customary for people living near the coasts to take children with deformities of their limbs out to the low-water level on the shore and there to bury the affected limbs under the wet sand for as long a period as possible between tides. This treatment was repeated until success was achieved. Whilst there is no scientific evidence for the success of this treatment the author has known people in the West Indies who have had personal experience of the treatment and claimed absolute success.

Certain ethnic or racial groups believe strongly in the health-giving properties of sea products. There are several forms in which some of the seaweeds are eaten as part of the routine diet. Laver bread made from seaweeds growing on the coast of the British Isles would be one example of a food product eaten as a dietary preparation for its rich mineral content and, in some cases its iodine content. The Japanese people are probably the main consumers of seaweed on a regular basis, believing strongly in its health-giving properties.

Of course just about all of us will eat seaweed products at some time or another, either as a dietary supplement in the form of kelp tablets, or more commonly, in the form of agar as used in thickeners for sauces, confectionery, salad dressings and ice creams.

Possibly the most well-known therapeutic application for seaweed would be the use of kelp in preparations for the treatment of goitre and thyroid dysfunctions. As will be seen later in this chapter, however, seaweeds possess many more therapeutic properties as well.

Indirectly even the consumption of ordinary fish has therapeutic implications. One of the reasons for the use of steamed or boiled fish in the diet fed to patients recovering from operations on the digestive system is that fish provides a more easily digested form of protein than do meat or dairy products. It is also high in nutritional value.

There are of course other applications of fish products more directly associated with their therapeutic properties. One common example is the use of cod or halibut liver oil in capsulated form as a source of vitamins A and D.

Turning to shellfish (but ignoring the alleged physiological effect of oysters combined with alcohol!), it has been recorded that, prior to the introduction of Western-style foods to some of the Polynesian races, the incidence of certain arthritic disorders was significantly less than it became when these people adopted the Western-style, processed food diet. The main significance of this observation is that the original diet of these Polynesian people comprised a high proportion of raw shellfish. The significance of the raw shellfish diet, (as opposed to the raw wetfish diet of the Japanese people), should not be overlooked when considering the product which forms the main subject for this book.

The Sea in Research and Pharmacology

The logical basis of utilizing the sea for the benefit of both medical research and treatment has been recognized for many years and has been studied by some marine research institutions since the late nineteen-thirties. However, it was only during the sixties that a significant effort to isolate and study biologically active substances with therapeutic potential was commenced. At the time of writing there is a considerable amount of such work in progress at universities and specialized research institutions all around the world. The reason for this growth in interest and action is the discovery that the seas and their inhabitants possess some unique, highly specific and highly potent substances previously unknown. It has been recognized that if some of these substances can be either obtained direct from the sea or synthetically prepared then some valuable new medical treatments will become available.

Another aspect of the intensified research programme has been the discovery that some marine creatures can function as excellent models in which to study the mechanism of glandular and hormonal reactions. The information so obtained can in many instances be related to that applicable to human physiology. For example, studies of reactions in specific marine organisms have contributed significantly to the understanding of osmo-regulation and kidney functions. Also studies on shark liver functions are promising a better understanding of some of the activities taking place in the human liver. Actually the shark is a most interesting creature, having existed in the same form for millions of years and generally being disease-free. Normally the shark only dies through old age or the activities of the human species, not through sickness.

In another field of study the interaction of neuro-transmitter systems in such creatures as the squid is leading to a fuller knowledge of brain mechanisms. This in turn should lead to improved facilities for dealing with neurological and psychiatric disorders in humans.

There are many other examples of the value of marine pharmacological and physiological research to both the understanding of complex human physiological reactions and the production of suitable treatments for the imbalances and disorders which affect them. Two such examples are the study of mucopoly-sacharrides in marine molluscs in relation to their influence on bronchial and pulmonary conditions in humans and the use of a species of crab to study the effects of cardiotoxic substances on heart function.

Whilst these research programmes are of great interest and will also yield information valuable for the future control of diseases of the body, it may be of more interest for the reader to hear of the developments which are actually yielding, or should soon yield, products which can be used to treat some of the more serious disorders from which we suffer.

In Japan an extract prepared from the Pacific oyster which is cultivated off the Sanriku coast is claimed to help diabetics by promoting the secretion of insulin. It is thought that it is the amino-acid Taurine naturally present in the oyster which is responsible for this beneficial property.

In France, investigation of a substance extracted from one of the red algae has indicated that in addition to possessing excellent and rather specific antibiotic properties, the preparation aids several healing and some dermatological problems.

Studies in the United States of America have resulted in the isolation of a substance from one of the many marine sponges which has antimicrobial activity being effective against gram-positive and gram-negative bacteria, and against yeasts and fungi.

Other researchers in the USA have investigated isolates from a whole range of marine plants and animals to produce cytotoxic extracts which have the property of being active against a specific group of micro-organisms. For example the substance would perhaps attack a fungal growth without adversely affecting other cells. A simple analogy to this specificity would be a weedkilling agent which could be applied to the lawn to kill undesirable weeds without having any adverse effect on the grass. One such substance which acts as a specific fungicide, Holotoxin, has been known for many years and is derived from a marine animal known as a sea-cucumber.

A considerable amount of research has been carried out, and still is being carried out, in the USA and elsewhere, on the screening of marine plants and animals for anti-cancer agents. Already some interesting substances with anti-cancer activity have been isolated from algae, sponges, jellyfish, corals, shellfish and other species.

Substances indicating cardio-vascular, immunological and anti-coagulant properties have been isolated from fish, algae and sponges and are currently undergoing investigation.

The ability of the alginates, a group of substances derived from seaweeds, to remove radioactive isotopes from the body without upsetting the balance of essential minerals has long been known. These alginates also have the ability to limit the uptake of the isotope strontium 87 from the gastro-intestinal tract in man. The value of such materials in diagnostic medicine using these isotopes can be appreciated.

Although there are many more examples of physiologically active extracts from marine organisms the few referred to above will at least give an indication of the potential value of these organisms in future medicine. It would hardly be appropriate, however, to complete this section of the book without including New Zealand green mussel extract. The effective use of this preparation for the relief of arthritic symptoms has taken place for over ten years. It has been shown to have both anti-inflammatory and gastro-protective properties with application in animal and human patients.

Farming the Sea

Some of the substances which are found in marine organisms and which have a valuable medicinal property will inevitably be produced synthetically. Once the identification and characterization of the active principle in the substance has been determined, modern chemical techniques will provide a method for synthesis of the active molecule and the requirement to use the plant or animal in which the activity was discovered will be ended.

There will, however, be instances where, because the activity of the organism depends on an interaction between two or more of its constituents or, because the active molecule is unstable in isolation, only the use of a preparation from the marine organism itself, in some cases even the whole organism, will be possible. In cases such as this it will be necessary to farm the sea actively to produce the new material for the product.

No doubt there are some exceptions to this statement, for instance it is not necessary to farm the sea to produce cod or halibut in order to obtain their liver oils. In the future this situation is not as likely to exist since many of the species needed will not be those harvested on a regular commercial basis, such as cod or halibut. Furthermore, conservation demands that heavy exploitation of natural marine resources such as occurs today will have to cease. Marine cultivation of appropriate species overcomes such problems.

Farming of the sea is not new. Under the modern title of 'aquaculture' farming of oysters, mussels, shrimps, prawns and various species of fish occurs quite extensively. One of the current developments is the farming of marine animals for the production of fish protein as a highly nutritious food for use in underdeveloped countries. A more financially orientated development is the production of shrimps and prawns to supplement declining catches from natural stocks.

There are several important features of marine farming which are not always appreciated by those not involved. It is these features which make the operation much more complex than it would appear and also, unfortunately, rather an expensive exercise.

Two main types of marine farming are in current use. One involves the use of tanks or ponds on shore through which sea water is pumped. The other requires the use of pens or other structures moored in the sea in or on which the farmed species is cultivated.

The shore tank system is particularly suited to the cultivation of algae, shrimps, prawns and some fish and shellfish. Some of the difficulties that arise with this type of operation occur because the stocks of the species involved are held in large populations in relatively confined spaces. Apart from the obvious problems of supplying adequate sea water to prevent de-oxygenation or the build-up of carbon dioxide and nitrogenous wastes, there is always a high risk of disease epidemics. Add to this the problems of artificially feeding the stock, predation on young by mature groups, maintenance of water quality and flow despite tidal variations, plus the very special habitat requirements of some species, and some appreciation of the difficulties involved is gained.

The system of cultivating the required species in the sea itself by use of pens or support structures removes some of the problems inherent in the shore tank system but unfortunately introduces others.

Naturally, whatever form of retaining system is used has to be able to withstand the fury of the elements. It is not always practical to make use of a sheltered spot due to the other requirements and restraints involved.

There are three main requirements for the offshore farm: adequate depth for the type of farming and structure involved; a reasonable tidal flow to give sufficient food and exchange of water; a location where the influence of drainage and rainwater run-off from adjacent land will not pollute the cultures. Having established these conditions, the next consideration is to have the farm located where it is practical to have staff on hand to work it and where it is not too far for the produce to be taken to where it will be utilized.

A less obvious problem with offshore farming is the environmental one. Argument is centred around the unsightliness of any moored structures in coastal waters (other than normal boats), commercial usage of a publicly owned natural resource and possible imbalance of the local ecology through concentration of a particular species.

It will be obvious that pollution of marine farm waters is a very important matter to consider. The effects of pollutants will naturally vary according to their type and concentration, but also according to the particular species being cultivated. For instance the presence of a level of arsenic or cynanide in sea water which would readily kill off a whole population of fish or crustaceans may have no effect on some molluscan shellfish provided it does not continue for more than a few days. This is because the shellfish would, upon detecting the alien substance in the water, immediately shut their shells and cease to filter or feed until all was well again. The main result of this would probably only be a weight loss. In other circumstances, however, it could be that a low level of a contaminant insufficient to kill fish or annoy the shellfish could be concentrated by the natural feeding process of the shellfish to a level dangerous to humans.

The reader will now understand that there are many and varied possibilities for problems in this area. Some contaminants are happily tolerated by marine species but seriously affect the human consuming them. Others directly affect the farmed species. Either way the marine farm suffers.

With specific regard to the cultivation of molluscan shellfish such as the mussel there are a few principal types of polluting effect to be guarded against. The most common of these is pollution by undesirable microbiological organisms likely to be present in domestic sewage discharges. Some pathogenic organisms are capable of fairly long-term survival in sea water despite their natural habitat being the human or animal body. Fortunately this type of polluting effect is easily detected and can be eliminated by a process of 'depuration'. This involves relaying the affected shellfish in clean or sterilized sea water for some forty-eight hours during which time they will purge themselves of the unwanted bacteria.

Next on the list of common pollutants come chemicals, in particular certain metal elements such as mercury, cadmium and lead. Whilst the presence of these contaminants is easily detected, they are not removed in the depuration process, being generally absorbed in the fatty content of the shellfish. Where this type of contaminant is present as a result of the discharge of industrial wastes to the sea, there is a distinct risk to the consumer. However, there are instances where the contaminants are present as a result of their natural presence in the waters. This may be a result of natural mineral deposits or volcanic activity. In such cases it does not always follow that a hazard exists.

Radioactive contamination of foods is a problem of our times and applies as much to marine species as to any other. Careful siting of the marine farm should preclude this risk. Again, whilst it is easy enough to detect this type of pollutant, it is not removable by current cleansing processes.

Whilst most of the polluting influences described above can be avoided by careful location of the marine farm site there is another source of contamination which cannot really be guarded against, and which should be monitored. This is contamination by toxins contained quite naturally in certain types of algae. These algae, which are usually only present at certain times of the year, can be filtered from the sea water by shellfish, thus transferring the toxins to the shellfish itself.

This phenomenon has been understood for many years and has been a frequent problem in the northern hemisphere. One of the better-known forms of this algal contamination in the northern hemisphere is known as 'red tide', caused by marine blooms of a dinoflagellate which turn the sea quite red in colour. In the southern hemisphere the problem has been very rare but there is evidence of the presence in New Zealand waters of some forms of algae known to contain specific toxins. Certainly it is no longer correct to assume that New Zealand green mussels will not contain toxins even though for most of the time they will not.

It is for the above reasons that the mussel extract forming the subject of this book is put through such a rigid quality control programme.

If all these problems discussed above are satisfactorily resolved, then the offshore marine farmer has only a few more naturally occurring problems to contend with. For example, in the cultivation of some shellfish it is common for heavy predation by fish to take place at certain times in the annual biological cycle. This could be prevented by suspending netting around the farm to preclude entry by predators. Unfortunately, this has two disadvantages. One of these is the rapid fouling of the net by marine growths which slow down or prevent the flow of water and food through the farm. The other is that fish will become stuck by their gills in the net, die and putrify, thus polluting the water around the farm. Of course there are solutions to these problems and at any rate they do not always occur in the first place. It is, however, advantageous to be aware of the possibility.

The Farming of the Green Mussel (*Perna canaliculus*)

There are two principal systems of farm cultivation of the New

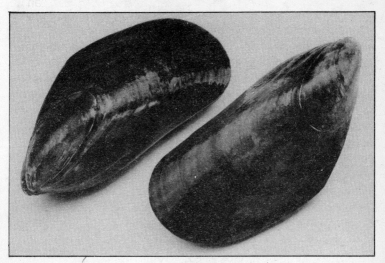

Figure 2. New Zealand green mussels (*Perna canaliculus*).

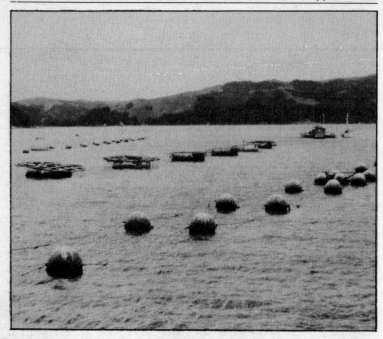

Figure 3.   Long lines and pontoons on a New Zealand green mussel farm

Zealand green mussel. (See Fig. 2.) *Perna canaliculus,* both of which are based on the vertical suspension of ropes holding the mussels. One of the systems involves the use of rafts or pontoons (see Fig. 3), from which the ropes of mussels are suspended. A similar system has been in use in Spain for many years.

The other system utilizes 'long lines' (see Fig. 3). These are ropes or wires stretched horizontally along the surface of the sea between anchored buoys. Other small buoys are attached to these long lines at intervals to hold them up as the weight of the growing mussels increases. The vertical ropes holding the mussels are suspended from the long lines at intervals of about one metre.

Both systems have advantages and disadvantages. For instance the pontoon system is the easier to work with when attaching ropes or 'thinning out' ropes. On the other hand, long lines tend to retain a mature crop in times of heavy weather more efficiently than do pontoons, due to their easier motion in a seaway.

Although it is possible to cultivate the larvae and very young mussels in a marine hatchery, it is not, under current circumstances, practical or economical to do so. The system currently in use in New Zealand for obtaining young seed stocks of mussels (called 'spat'), employs the use of special 'spat' collecting long line farms in the country's west-coast harbours. Here settlement of seed mussels is usually heavy. However, these areas are not suitable for rearing these seed mussels through to the adult stage.

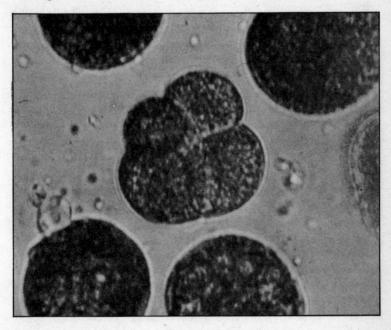

Figure 4a. The egg of the New Zealand green mussel undergoing cell division after fertilization

For readers unfamiliar with the life cycle of the mussel, a brief description follows.

At the appropriate time of year (around June/July for *Perna canaliculus*), the female mussel (orange-coloured) begins to discharge her eggs. An adult female may discharge up to 30 million eggs in one spawning. This action stimulates the male mussel (creamy white) to release millions of sperms.

Somehow the tadpole-like sperm manage to locate an egg and fertilize it by penetrating the egg wall. During the forty-eight hours following fertilization the egg undergoes normal cell division, finally becoming a free-swimming veliger. The larval form of the mussel remains free-swimming amongst the plankton for about three weeks, during which time it filters microscopic plant cells for food and develops the shell needed for protection and survival.

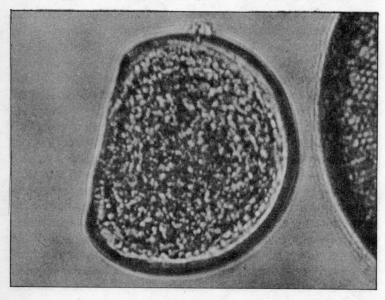

Figure 4b.   The free-swimming larval stage of the New Zealand green mussel

At about 3-4 weeks the mussel larvae has attained a size of about ¼ mm across the shell and is seeking a firm base such as a rock, wooden post or hanging rope on which to settle. Having found a suitably secure home the larvae anchors itself strongly with a thread called a 'byssus' and gives up the free-swimming life. It is now a sedentary organism and if undisturbed, will rapidly adopt the shape, then the colouring, of the adult mussel. Under natural conditions the green mussel could be expected to grow steadily for about seven or eight years and to attain a shell size of some 175-180 mm.

In the process of farm cultivation of the green mussel the 3-4-week-old larvae are allowed to settle on ropes which are left undisturbed for a further four to five weeks to allow the young mussels to grow to about 5 mm and become quite settled with their rope home.

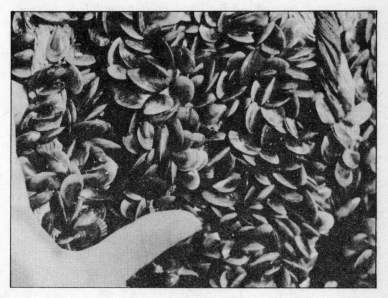

Figure 4c.   Young (seed) green mussels growing on the ropes they were caught on and ready for transplanting

At this point the ropes, plus seed mussels, are transferred to the growing area farms on the east coast of the North Island and also in the 'Sounds' areas of the South Island to be thinned out, reseeded and allowed to grow for some eighteen to twenty-four months before being harvested for use. At the harvest time the mussels should easily exceed 10 cm in length.

There is nothing that can be deemed truly artificial in the marine cultivation of New Zeland green mussels. The reason for their more rapid growth and better condition than would normally occur is merely that they are placed in the optimum conditions for food supply and growth. The vertical suspension system allows the maximum utilization of the water column, tidal stream, etc., and the thinning and appropriate seeding levels for the ropes balances competition for food to a manageable level. In natural settlement conditions it is entirely a matter of the 'survival of the fittest'!

2

The Disease

It would hardly seem appropriate to have a book on the subject of a treatment for arthritic disorders without some reference to the disease itself. In this chapter some of the more commonly experienced forms of rheumatism and arthritis are described. Also, some of the difficulties facing the rheumatologist who is attempting to assess the effect of treatment on the disease by means of clinical trials are discussed.

Arthritic disorders of one kind or another have always plagued mankind and animals. Evidence of arthritic influences has been observed in fossilized and prehistoric animal skeletons and in mummified human corpses. It is quite possible that some forms of the disease may even be evolutionary. For example, the gradual stiffening up, shrinkage and loss of mobility in elderly people and animals could well be a natural development designed to preclude members of a species from dominating beyond the term of their capacity to do so effectively.

Undoubtedly some forms of the disease are the result of normal wear and tear on body structure. However, other forms have no connection with these natural processes whatsoever. This is supported by the fact that babies and young children may suffer from a form of juvenile arthritis known as Still's disease. There are also forms of arthritis which are of a constant and lasting nature whilst some, such as bursitis, housemaid's knee and tennis elbow, may be of a transient nature.

What Causes Arthritis?

It is necessary here to differentiate between the various types of the disease. For instance, it is known that osteo-arthrosis is a condition resulting from the natural ageing and wearing processes in the joints. On the other hand, whilst much is known about rheumatoid arthritis and its control, the cause of this disorder remains, as yet, unknown.

It will probably be more helpful to deal with the curative or influential factors in the different forms of the disease as each one is addressed.

Osteo-Arthrosis

This disorder is also commonly known as osteo-arthritis. However, the term 'itis' is usually reserved for diseases of an inflammatory nature and it is more correctly described by the term arthrosis.

As the name suggests osteo-arthrosis is a disease associated with the bone structure. It may be described in general terms as a degenerative disease, the degenerative factor being associated with the articular cartilage and joint surfaces.

Although there are several theories suggesting the cause of degeneration in joints, possibly the most favoured theory relates to the effect of continual impact forces on the articular cartilage. To take the hip joint as an example, the effect of continually jarring the joint in some forms of athletics could be to gradually reduce the ability of the articular cartilage to absorb shock. In time, destruction of the cartilage could occur with corresponding breakdown of joint surfaces. This theory does explain the incidence of osteo-arthrosis in overweight people and athletes where normal ageing has not been the cause.

Another manifestation of osteo-arthrosis is often quite visible in the form of knobbly lumps or spurs on the finger joints. These spurs are caused by the joints attempting to heal themselves by forming new cartilage which unfortunately tends to form hard knobs. These knobs later become bony themselves and of course severely restrict movement of the joint.

All the joints in the body may be affected by osteo-arthrosis. It is more commonly experienced in the toes, fingers, knees, hip, spine and neck.

Apart from taking care not to subject our joints unnecessarily to impact or to overload the weight-bearing ones by being consistently overweight there is little we can do to change the course of this disease for which we are all potential victims.

Rheumatoid Arthritis

In contrast to osteo-arthrosis, rheumatoid arthritis is an inflammatory disease and, although involved with joints, is not degenerative. This disorder is created when inflammation affects the linings of joints. Just as inflammation of the skin caused by a sting or wound infection causes swelling, heat and pain, so too does inflammation of the joint linings. However, it does not require much imagination to see that in the case of joint linings suffering inflammation, movement of the joint would be at least rather painful and possibly severely restricted.

Rheumatoid arthritis is not a condition restricted to the elderly or athletes. It has no age barriers and can even affect young children. For a reason which would certainly seem to be associated with female hormones the disease is much more common in women than in men. The severity of rheumatoid arthritis can vary from the case of a person who merely suffers mild pain and stiffness in certain joints for a short period first thing in the morning, to the case where the person is bedridden, has distorted limbs and has to be maintained on constant drug therapy just to try to control the situation.

The cause of rheumatoid arthritis is not yet known although there are several theories proposed. It would be out of context and beyond the scope of this book to deal with all the theories available. However, the main ones currently offered in explanation are briefly outlined here.

One theory is based on the principle of the body's natural immune response system. It is suggested that the natural defence mechanism of the body recognizes some component of the joint lining (called the synovium) as an enemy and therefore attacks it. When an immunological attack is taking place it is normally accompanied by an inflammatory reaction.

Another suggestion is that the inflammation in the joint is the result of a persistent infection. The organism responsible for such infection has not yet been determined but there are other cases of inflammatory conditions being caused by infection of this type.

Possibly the most recent suggestion for the cause is related to a group of substances known as prostaglandins. These are a special class of unsaturated fatty acids which have a high level of physiological activity. They are involved in various bodily functions including ovulation, maintenance of blood pressure, smooth muscle stimulation, etc. It is known that inhibition of the synthesis of certain prostaglandins in the body is affected by some of the anti-inflammatory drugs and, incidentally also by the mussel extract. Quite possibly then these prostaglandins are influential in the inflammatory processes involved in rheumatoid arthritis. Some support is lent to this hypothesis by the fact that rheumatoid arthritis symptoms may disappear in women during pregnancy and at menopause when hormonal changes occur.

Gout
This is a form of arthritis in which extremely painful inflammatory attacks can occur as result of the precipitation of uric acid crystals from the blood. It usually affects the wrists, knees or feet, being most common probably in the joints of the big toe. In contrast to rheumatoid arthritis, gout is more commonly found in men than in women. When it does occur in women it is usually in the post-menopausal phase of life.

Traditionally the cause of gout has been linked to high living. This may well be true since the consumption of large, rich meals accompanied by plenty of alcohol would stimulate production of uric acid and concurrently inhibit the disposal of it by the kidneys. However, many gout sufferers lead a very moderate lifestyle and suffer the disorder due to some defect in their system which allows the build-up of uric acid in the bloodstream to reach a level at which its solubility is exceeded and it therefore crystallizes out. The pain is caused by the physical presence of the acid crystals in the joint lining.

Ankylosing Spondylitis

This is a form of arthritis in which an inflammatory condition in the joints of the spine creates bony growths which actually connect up separate joints to one another. The result is that the spine becomes rigid and the unfortunate sufferer is severely restricted in movement.

This condition is not so rare as might be imagined. In fact it is a common cause of back problems in young men in their twenties. As with gouty arthritis the condition is much more prevalent in men than in women. The cause of the initial inflammatory response is not known but the progress and mechanism of the disorder resulting from it are well documented. Fortunately, in many cases it disappears after a few years and, apart from some occasional backache, the person feels quite well again.

Carpal Tunnel Syndrome

Another reasonably common form of arthritis, carpal tunnel syndrome, involves inflammation of the lining of the carpal tunnel in the wrist which, due to the lack of space in the tunnel, creates pressure on the tendons and median nerve which pass through it. This in turn causes paralysis in the fingers and pain in the hand and arm. The condition is more common in women than in men, in particular during pregnancy and at the menopause.

Lumbago or Fibrositis

These terms are generally used to describe non-specific back or neck pains. In the case of lumbago it is the lower back or 'lumbar' region which is involved. The conditions can occur in anyone and are sometimes related to heavy lifting, back posture, sleeping with a pillow at the wrong height and so on. The cause is not known but is probably associated with some degeneration of spinal cartilage. An unfortunate side-effect of the condition is that there is no physical manifestation of the problem, and the idea that someone is merely shirking duties by claiming to have back troubles can be psychologically upsetting to the genuine sufferer.

Bursitis

The two most common occurrences of this disorder are in the form of 'housemaid's knee' and bursitis of the shoulder. The pain arises due to inflammation of the bursae, which are specially lined, closed sacs designed to lubricate the areas where muscles rub against joints. In the case of 'housemaid's knee' it is the prolonged kneeling which creates pressure on the bursae and results in inflammation. Where the shoulder is involved, it is inflammation of the tunnel through which the tendons pass which causes the problem. This is why, only when the arm is in certain positions, pain is experienced because the bursae are only compressed in the tunnel at certain stages of movement.

Bursitis is not the cause of 'frozen shoulder', which is a different condition altogether, described in medical terms as 'capsulitis'. This is a disorder previously associated with middle and old age.

Tennis Elbow

This condition could equally well be called 'Golfers' Elbow' since the effect is the same. The muscles on the opposite side of the joint to each other are involved in the two named conditions. Again the pain, swelling and restriction of movement are the result of inflammation. These forms of arthritis which can of course be caused by activities other than those of tennis or golf are basically self-induced due to repeated extension and contraction of the muscles.

Psoriatic Arthritis

This is a form of the disease in which two separate conditions exist simultaneously. The psoriasis is a skin condition in which patches of red, flaky skin appear, most frequently in areas such as the scalp, elbow and knees. It often coincides with rheumatoid arthritis and opinions differ as to whether the two conditions are actually associated or merely coincidental. There is evidence to suggest that the condition may involve a hereditary factor. Psoriatic arthritis should not be confused with psoriatic arthropathy which is a different disease altogether. In this condition it is usually the fingertip joints which become inflamed with the psoriasis affecting the fingernails.

Reiter's Disease

This is a form of arthritis which was long thought to be a direct result of venereal disease. There is evidence to support the theory that venereal disease can lead to an attack of Reiter's disease. However, it is equally evident that it can be caused by other conditions, such as infectious dysentery.

This is a particularly unpleasant form of arthritis usually affecting young adults. Apart from the normal pain associated with an inflammatory condition the sufferer may also experience conjunctivitis in both eyes, considerable discomfort in passing urine, skin rash and ulcers. Fortunately the condition responds well to proper treatment.

Still's Disease

As was mentioned earlier in this chapter, arthritis can even strike in young children. In general terms Still's disease is a form of rheumatoid arthritis in children. Fortunately the incidence of this disorder is fairly rare and also the condition is often temporary. More girls than boys tend to be affected and there is opinion that it may have a hereditary element.

It is particularly distressing to see otherwise healthy children suffering Still's disease at the age when they should have maximum mobility and freedom from the worries of adult life, and when of course they are still undergoing structural development. On the brighter side, however, the majority of children affected by this form of arthritis grow out of it.

Rheumatic Fever

This is a condition of known cause and, happily, through the ability to control the cause, of diminishing occurrence. The disease is caused by a particular bacteria called *Streptococcus*, though it does not follow that a streptococcal infection will result in rheumatic fever. The main symptoms of the disease are combined fever and inflamed joints and it is, or was, most common in children. Whilst there are lasting effects in some cases, in particular if the heart muscle has been involved, these are quite controllable with medical supervision.

In the developed countries where effective hygiene codes are observed, rheumatic fever has almost disappeared. As progress is made with the introduction of better sanitation and hygiene in underdeveloped regions so too will microbiologically influenced diseases like rheumatic fever decline.

Factors which can Influence Arthritis

It is well known that factors not directly related to a particular disorder can significantly influence its course and, in some instances, possibly even its onset. For example, whilst it is appreciated that the common cold cannot be caught simply by being cold and wet there can be little doubt that exposure to such conditions would aggravate the situation providing that the cold virus were present. If a person is cold, wet and uncomfortable it is to be expected that their resistance to infection or the effects of infection would be lowered. It is also true of course that psychological influences can significantly affect the course of a disease.

Two of the main factors known or thought to influence arthritic disorders are stress and diet. These are discussed below.

Stress

Stress influences both humans and animals. It takes many forms and its effects are widespread. In the author's opinion, which it must be explained is based on experience only and not on any medical knowledge or training, stress is probably the most significant factor influencing arthritic sufferers. Whether stress factors can be involved in actually causing some forms of arthritis is not known, but it is certain that they can initiate regression and recurrence in the disease. Rheumatoid arthritis is a disease which is subject to natural remission. How many people, after having experienced natural remission have found that their arthritic condition has suddenly returned following a period of anxiety?

It is not only sad or unpleasant occurrences that cause the physiological changes associated with stress. Emotions such as excessive happiness or excitement create a stress factor too. It is probably fair to say, however, that more stress conditions are associated with worry and unhappy events than with excessive joy.

Climatic conditions can play a stressful as well as a physical role in their influence on people. The depression created by a long period of bad weather, anger at unseasonal conditions interfering with holiday plans, anxiety about possible storm damage occurring to one's home; all are weather-influenced stress situations outside the more usual ones of direct discomfort due to cold, heat or damp. Excessive heat is just as much a stress factor as is excessive cold, a point sometimes not appreciated by arthritics living in cold areas and wishing that they could move to the tropics!

Environmental circumstances have come to play a more significant part in creating stress conditions in recent years. For example people have been housed in high-rise flats where, apart from the isolation associated with these dwellings, they are in an unfamiliar area. It would be of considerable interest to have a statistical analysis carried out on the effect of such moves on arthritic complaints.

There is more than one way in which stress can influence disease processes. It can act to lower a person's resistance to pain, which in turn creates more stress and begins a downward spiral. It may act to influence hormonal activity to the extent that the body's physiology is changed.

To clarify this a little, the body reacts to a disease or emotion by inducing chemical changes. In some instances the adoptive powers will involve the development of antibodies to combat a specific antigen. In other instances, for example fright or anger, it may be a hormonal stimulation such as the release of cortisone by the adrenal gland. These adoptive processes are generally involuntary, that is the person or animal involved does not make a conscious effort to invoke them. However, under stress conditions it is possible that the processes are influenced in a manner which makes resistance to the disease condition less effective. In the case of hormonal influences it is probable that this is due to a change in the activity of the hormones and not to any difference in the concentration or amount of hormones present.

As stress factors can influence hormonal activities which in turn control the functioning of our bodies it is not difficult to appreciate the significant role these emotions play in our well-being.

Diet

The influence of diet on arthritic conditions has received a considerable amount of attention. There are so many foods claimed to be harmful in different schools of thought that there would be little left to eat if all were taken seriously. As with many things, it is a case of 'One man's meat is another man's poison.'

It is quite reasonable to assume that diet will significantly influence the physiological activities of the body. Just what activities occur will depend on the digestion and assimilation of the foods concerned. Assimilation is the key factor because if the results of digestion are not assimilated then no physiological processes will take place.

Digestion (or indigestion) can be very influential on the symptoms of arthritis. It may well be that the people who claim that red meat or 'acidic' fruits are bad for arthritis are actually being influenced by adverse digestive processes. In turn these processes will cause discomfort and possibly even pain and will tend to aggravate any other complaint suffered by these people. Indirectly of course these foods would be bad for those concerned since they aggravate the arthritis by a stress factor rather than by a direct biochemical reaction.

Certain dietary recommendations can reasonably be made, both for control of the disease and as prophylactic measures. For instance it would seem acceptable that a balanced diet of fresh vegetables, seafoods, dairy produce, some meats (but particularly liver and kidneys) is beneficial. Provided the essential nutrients are assimilated, then the elements necessary for a healthy metabolism are provided to the system.

A complication has been introduced into the availability of a good, healthy balanced diet in recent years by the treatment of meat animals and crops for disease whilst growing. Unfortunately some of the injections, sprays and powder dustings can carry right through to the consumer. Though there is no definite chemical evidence to associate these substances with arthritic disorders it is reasonable to suggest that they would not be helpful.

Many bodily disorders are the result of a breakdown in metabolic processes. These are controlled by chemical stimuli which in turn are triggered by enzymes derived from nutrition. If the source and utilization of nutrition are appropriate then such disorders should be avoided. Also, the better nourished, fitter and physiologically sound·the body is, the more able it is to resist malfunction.

The Assessment of New Treatments

New and varied treatments are constantly being presented for arthritic diseases. The rheumatologist needs to be satisfied that the new treatments are effective and do not have such unpleasant side-effects that they are unsafe to use. For this reason trials are designed to assess the effects of the treatments on patients under carefully controlled clinical conditions. The most commonly used procedure for this exercise is known as a 'Double Blind Trial'. It is so designed that half of a group of patients receive the test substance whilst the other half receive a preparation of similar appearance, odour, etc., but which has no pharmacological activity (called a placebo). Neither the doctor administrating the trial nor the patient taking part is aware of who is receiving which substance until after the trial has been completed. This method rules out or minimizes the probability of the doctor or patient being psychologically influenced.

Unfortunately there are some factors beyond clinical control which can significantly influence the trial results, particularly in the case of trials involving arthritic patients. Whilst the existence of these factors is known to doctors conducting clinical trials, it is not always possible for the doctor to be aware that they are actually taking place.

One of the most influential factors is created by the fact that most trials involving arthritic patients need to employ outpatients as trial subjects. The result of this can be a high drop-out rate due perhaps to difficulties in getting to the hospital for checks, caused by bad weather, transport strikes and so on.

Another factor can be the adverse effect on a patient who has had to wait for a long time in a cold or uncomfortable outpatient waiting room. Apart from the reluctance to continue attending for trial purposes there can also be a stress factor created by the prolonged wait or the discomfort.

The attitude of the patient to the doctor can also be a significant factor in the demonstrative side of trial assessments. There can be a considerable difference in both the verbal answers to questions and the effort put into the physical exercises used to measure response to treatment depending on whether the patient likes the physician and wants to do well for him or her, or is feeling antagonistic and performs accordingly.

It hardly needs mentioning that the introduction of a stress situation at home or work which is unrelated to, but, occurring during the trial can have a significant influence on patient response to the test medication.

It is very easy to criticize trial procedures and not nearly so easy to suggest alternatives which will cover all the points raised. This section of the book has not been intended as destructive criticism at all. Its purpose has been to indicate that where human trial subjects are involved the results of even well-designed trials may be influenced by issues outside the trial parameters.

3

The Mussel Extract Treatment

The Discovery

There have been varying reports of the original discovery of the anti-arthritic properties of the New Zealand green mussel. One report claims that the discovery occurred as a result of investigative work in the field of nutrition by an American systems control engineer named Arthur Eriksen. Apparently the connection between the nutritive and anti-arthritic properties resulted from the experiences of friends of Mr Eriksen who found that their arthritic problems had disappared after eating a 'nutrient extract' of the mussel which he had prepared.

Another report based the discovery on research which was involved with the investigation of potential anti-cancer agents derived from marine organisms. During the nineteen-sixties and seventies a considerable amount of funding was directed towards the search for anti-cancer agents in natural substances. Some of this funding was directed towards marine research at US universities equipped to carry out such specialized work. One of the shellfish to be screened in this programme was apparently the New Zealand green mussel, *Perna canaliculus*, and, whilst no anti-cancer activity was noted, an anti-inflammatory activity was.

Some credence may be attributed to this report on the basis that earlier research had established biological activity against tumours and a type of leukaemia (in mice) which originated in the shellfish *Mercenaria mercenaria*. This shellfish is a clam which is a bivalve mollusc, as is the mussel. It is not difficult to imagine the degree of enthusiasm with which the screening of other molluscan shellfish would have been conducted following such a finding.

Whatever the true origin of the discovery may be, it is certain that it was made in the United States and passed on to New Zealand, because the mussel *Perna canaliculus* is both indigenous and peculiar to that country. The New Zealand investigations and research began in 1973 and led to the worldwide distribution of the product in a form suitable for use by both human and animal subjects.

The Production and Chemistry of New Zealand Green Mussel Extract

The extract is produced at a factory in the western part of Auckland City, New Zealand. However, the mussels which are used in the preparation of the extract are selected from marine farms in both the north and south islands of the country. It will be seen as this chapter proceeds that the geographical distribution of the mussel cultivation areas plays a vitally important part in the production of an effective and safe product.

Selecting the Mussels

The mussels used in the preparation of the mussel extract product which is the subject of this book are selected on the basis of their condition in relation to gonad development, their quality in relation to freedom from chemical and microbiological contaminants and their safety in relation to the absence of marine toxins of the types causing either diarrhetic or paralytic shellfish poisoning. Having established that the mussels are satisfactory in these respects, they are assayed for 'activity' to see that they will be effective. It does not follow that satisfactory condition and quality automatically guarantee 'activity'.

It must be pointed out here, in support of statements made elsewhere in this book about possible dangers associated with imitation products, that the testing of the shellfish to satisfy all of the above requirements is essential to the production of a safe product. To carry out this procedure, samples of mussels from the different areas of marine cultivation in New Zealand are tested before harvesting begins. Upon satisfactory results being achieved the mussels are harvested and transported in a cool (but not refrigerated), covered environment to the processing factory as quickly as possible. At the factory the mussels are processed to a patented method described briefly below.

It was mentioned earlier that the variation in geographical situations of the mussel cultivation areas was important in relation to the production of a safe and effective product. This is because the mussels are only in a usable condition for a certain period of the year. There are two reasons for this, one being related to the condition and 'activity level' of the mussels and the other related to possible contamination by marine algae which introduce the toxic factors mentioned earlier. Both causes are related to seawater temperatures and weather patterns. They are not accurately predictable, hence the need for constant testing.

Fortunately the distribution of the cultivation areas in New Zealand is such that it has proved to be extremely unlikely that all mussels would be in a non-usable condition at the same time. It is also evident that some regions are more likely to suffer undesirable influences than others. It is attention to these matters involving constant laboratory testing and monitoring that ensures the use of suitable mussels for the process.

The Production of Mussel Extract

The mussel extract is produced under licence to a patented method. The method was patented as a result of research in Japan which developed the process to ensure that the 'activity' present in the shellfish was not destroyed in the processing phase of the operation. Only one company is licensed to use this method of production. This is another reason for exercising caution when selecting the product to try.

The method involves the extraction of that portion of the shellfish containing the 'activity'. This is achieved by a centrifugal method.

The resultant product of this exercise is a rich liquid which, after treatment to stabilize its activity level, is freeze-dried to produce a cream-coloured biscuit.

The process of freeze-drying is important in that it reduces the moisture content of the product to less than 3 per cent by weight. When this has been done the product is also stable with regard to microbiological decomposition, hydrolysis and such. However, it is frequently said that freeze-drying is simply the removal of water without the use of excessive heat to boil it off. This is not accurate and a brief explanation of why it is not seems warranted.

Freeze-drying really means the process of removing moisture by vacuum distillation. The benefit of the vacuum distillation is that it allows moisture to be distilled (boiled off) with the product at low temperatures, so that protein substances remain intact instead of being denatured and rendered inactive.

During the freeze-drying process it is important that the moisture in the product, which is in the frozen state at the start of the programme, goes direct from solid (ice) to vapour in one stage without passing through the liquid (water) phase.

To achieve this the product is subject to the combined effect of vacuum, refrigeration and heating. If these are not carefully controlled, and the internal product temperature-monitored, it is quite possible for processes to occur within the protein molecules which render them inactive as proteins. Indeed, subjecting samples of the same liquid extract to different freeze-drying techniques can yield substances with quite different characteristics.

Following freeze-drying, the product, in biscuit form, is subjected to a three-stage disintegration process which yields the fine power, used as it is — in powder form — or in capsules or tablets.

Quality Control

At all stages from fresh mussel to finished, capsulated product sampling and constant monitoring of the product takes place. It is as necessary to establish that secondary contamination of the product during its progress through the factory does not occur as it is to ensure that the raw material is free from contamination.

The tests applied relate to the basic chemical composition of the product, specific contaminants such as mercury, cadmium, zinc and lead, microbiological contaminants from human or animal sources and, of course, the retention of the product 'activity'.

Five laboratories are involved in this work: two separate laboratories at the factory itself; one independent commercial laboratory in New Zealand (for independent certification); one Government laboratory in Australia; and one research laboratory in Japan.

The Chemistry of the Extract

The figures given in Table 2 indicate the basic composition of New Zealand green mussel extract as produced by the patent method referred to earlier. Although there are of course differences in the expanded analysis of the product from that which would be obtained from other molluscan shellfish, there is nothing as yet which can be directly attributable to the pharmacological activity of the product. This is not at all surprising and is explained below. First, however, a few observations on the basic analysis as shown in Table 2 may be of interest.

The protein level may not appear to be particularly high but it must be remembered that it is not always the amount of a substance that creates an effect but rather the composition. Proteins are highly complex molecules made up of individual amino acids in a similar way to that in which words are made up of the letters of the alphabet. In the very same way it cannot be assumed that a list of the amino acids, or even their relative quantities, indicates anything definite about a substance. For example if we take the individual letters M, A, T and E, to represent just four amino acids it can be seen immediately that we have the possibility of four completely different proteins analogous to the words MEAT, MATE, TEAM and TAME. Each of the four proteins has the same amino acid analysis but would be a totally different compound.

It is worth remembering that some of the most lethal poisons are proteins made up of the same amino acids as the favourite fish we eat with valued nutritional benefit! Fortunately the arrangement of the acids and their bonding within the protein compound is different, hence the pharmacological effect.

Table 2. New Zealand Mussel Extract Basic Composition

Minerals	Composition 5 g/100g
Sodium	
Potassium	1
	mg/100g
Magnesium	350
Calcium	500
Iron	30
Zinc	5
Manganese	1
Copper	1
Nickel	0.4
Cadmium	0.4
Lead	0.4
Mercury	0.01
Vitamins	
B1	0 – 0.2
B2	0 – 0.2
B3	0 – 0.4
B6	0 – 0.2
B12	0 – 0.2
C	0 – 0.2
D3	0 – 0.3
E	0 – 0.2
	g/100g
Protein (N × 6.25)	40 – 50

	Composition g/100g
Lipids	15 – 20
Cholesterol	0.1 – 0.2
Carbohydrate (by diff)	5 – 15
Mineral ash	20 – 30
Moisture Less than	3
Calorie value	ca 400 calories/100g

Amino Acids	g/100g
Cysteic acid	2.3
Aspartic acid	3.2
Threonine	1.4
Serine	1.5
Glutamic acid	4.0
Proline	1.2
Glycine	4.0
Alanine	1.7
Cysteine	0.2
Valine	1.5
Methionine	0.8
Iso-Leucine	1.4
Leucine	2.1
Tyrosine	1.2
Phenylalanine	1.3
Lysine	2.7
Histidine	0.7
Arginine	2.5

Because the mussels live in sea water they contain an excellent mineral balance. The sea contains all the minerals known to man. Some of these are shown in the mussel extract analysis in Table 2, though these are only the ones present at the higher concentrations. Mussels, in common with other filter feeding molluscan shellfish, have the ability to concentrate minerals or other substances present in the sea water in which they live. It is quite natural to find higher levels of mineral elements present in the shellfish than those of the surrounding waters. Provided that the elements are useful to the human body and not toxic, then the mussels, and the mussel extract, provide an excellent balanced mineral supplement.

The level of lipids (fats and oils) present in the extract varies according to that of the shellfish used. This in turn varies during the season but is generally at its highest level when the shellfish are in their peak condition. Being marine lipids the greater proportion are of the polyunsaturated groups and do not present problems such as those generally associated with cholesterol. In fact there is a school of thought which actually advocates the use of marine lipids in the form of processed fish oils, for the treatment and prevention of such disorders as arteriosclerosis. This is not to suggest that the mussel extract product has any benefit in this direction whatsoever, but merely to indicate that the use of some fish oils is considered to be therapeutic rather than detrimental to arterial and blood vessel functions.

Cholesterol itself is usually present at about 0.1 − 0.2 per cent, which is insignificant. Compare this level with that of an egg, which would average 0.5 - 0.6 per cent. It is easy to see that, on the basis of taking approximately 1g of mussel extract per day, the amount of cholesterol involved would be 1-2mg. Eating one average egg of about 50g weight per day would involve 250-300mg of cholesterol.

The vitamins shown in the analysis are all present naturally, that is to say they have not been added to the extract to supplement it. The amounts are low and the extract could not be considered to be a vitamin supplement. However, it is the author's opinion that vitamin supplements are often overloaded and wasteful. It is sound comment that, provided a reasonably balanced diet is consumed, the body needs no supplementary vitamins or, at best, only minimal quantities.

Which Part of the Extract Has the Therapeutic Properties?

The straight answer to this question is very short and simple: we don't know! It would not be fair to leave things at that, however, as a lot of work has been done to try to establish the identity of the 'active principle'.

Some readers might at this point be wondering how it is that, since the identity of the active principle (the therapeutic part) of this product is not yet known, it can be claimed, as it was earlier in this chapter, that the method of production allows the activity to remain at its original level and be stabilized. This is explained by the fact that laboratory methods to measure the degree of activity are available using special bio-assay techniques. These methods do not indicate what is causing the activity, merely that it is there.

Fractionation and biological testing are still proceeding on samples of mussel extract which are sent every month to research institutes specializing in this type of work. Eventually the answer will be established. At any rate, the work completed so far has upheld the view that the extract is of benefit in relieving the symptoms of arthritis, and has gone some way towards explaining why this should be, at least narrowing the field of investigation.

One line of research has shown quite definitely that the anti-inflammatory properties of the mussel extract can be linked to its protein content. Further expansion of this work indicated that the protein is in the water-soluble rather than the fat-soluble group and appears to be a high molecular weight compound. What this means is that the protein is not just a simple one but could well have complex radicals bonded to it. In this case it becomes a much more difficult exercise to isolate and identify it. Another aspect of this finding is that it suggests that the preparation of a synthetic substance of the same structure will be difficult.

Researchers adopting another approach found that the lipid fraction of the extract demonstrated a gastro-protective activity. This is a very valuable discovery since it suggests that the extract will not cause ulceration or haemorrhage of the stomach as happens with some commonly used drug therapies. Additionally it was found that if the extract was added to one of the drug treatments that did cause stomach damage it not only prevented or minimized the damage but also complemented the anti-inflammatory action of the drug.

The results of the two programmes just described certainly suggest that the extract should be used in its present form even should the active anti-inflammatory principle be isolated. The active principle, if used in isolation, could well cause side-effects similar to those of some of the drug treatments. It may indeed be the very fact that it is 'screened' within the bulk of the extract including the lipid fraction that prevents such effects.

In conclusion it may be said that the results of the research conducted between 1974 and 1985 indicate that the therapeutic properties of the extract are most probably associated with a high molecular weight protein possibly supplemented by activity in the lipid fraction of the extracts.

The research programmes that have been conducted to attempt to isolate and identify the therapeutic part of the mussel extract product are summarized in Chapter 4.

The Mussel Extract Treatment

A question frequently asked is, 'If this treatment from the sea is so marvellous, why is it not more widely advertised, and why doesn't everyone use or recommend it?' The question is a fair one and will be answered here.

There are two aspects to the answer to the first part of the question. First of all, the mussel extract is only marvellous for some people, good for others and not at all helpful to some. This is a common feature of all medication and it is true to say that there is no medication whatsoever that will help everyone. Furthermore, the mussel extract product is not a 'miracle cure'. It is as effective as most of the anti-arthritic drugs in use without the serious side-effects associated with those drugs.

Secondly the product is not registered as a 'drug'. It is the law of most countries nowadays that only products registered as 'drugs' (the therapeutic kind) may have advertising which makes or even infers therapeutic claims for their use. This is basically sound legislation designed to protect the public from fraudulent claims by unscrupulous operators. Before any therapeutic claims may be made for a 'drug' product it must be subjected to lengthy and expensive test procedures to establish that it works.

The mussel extract product has undergone most of the tests applied to drugs which establish that it works and is safe. It is, however, still classified as a 'health food' or 'food supplement'. Thus, although it is effective therapeutically it cannot yet be advertised as such. Progress towards registration of the product to allow advertising of its therapeutic properties is still being made.

It is normal practice to conduct trials with animal subjects under laboratory conditions in the investigation of any new therapeutic substances. Some of the trial work is designed to establish that the substance is safe for use with human subjects and some to attempt to establish information as to what physiological changes are being caused by its use. This work is essential and cannot be done without the aid of the animal subjects, normally laboratory-bred rats or mice. Clinical trials using human subjects complement this research and demonstrate the practical use of the substance under test. The information obtained from such research using the mussel extract as the test substance is the basis of this chapter. Detailed comment on each individual research programme follows in Chapter 4.

It has been the success of the mussel extract in relieving the symptoms of various forms of arthritis in people all around the world that has created the research interest in the product. Scientific institutions in many different countries, including New Zealand, Australia, Japan, the United Kingdom, the United States, Germany, Holland, Switzerland and France have all had a part in determining the facts which follow.

Frequently the research has been inspired as a result of a friend or relative of someone working at the hospital or research centre experiencing the beneficial results of the mussel extract capsules which were probably sent for them to try by a caring relative living in New Zealand. More recently, people visiting New Zealand on holiday have discovered the properties of the product for themselves and then reported their success to interested scientific friends back home. In other instances these visitors have acted as information gatherers for interested people back home by visiting the production factory in Auckland, New Zealand.

Using the Treatment

The treatment involves the regular taking on a daily basis of the mussel extract in capsule form. The fine powder yielded by the factory processing of the mussels is placed in hard gelatine capsules containing either 230mg net or 350mg net weight of extract per capsule. The usual dosage taken each day is either 5 of the 230mg or 3 of the 350mg capsules. The capsules should be taken with and not between meals to minimize the risk of indigestion. Whether the total daily dosage is taken with one meal or is spread over several meals does not appear to have any significant effect on the results obtained.

Quite naturally the first question most people ask is 'How long will it be before I feel any results?' The second question is usually 'Will I have to continue taking the capsules forever?' Although there are certain patterns of reaction to the product that have become evident from trial work and general experience over the ten years of widespread use, it must be stressed that people react individually to all medication. Therefore, whereas one person may respond to a particular treatment within a day or two, another may take weeks to respond or not even respond at all.

In general, people using the mussel extract have begun to notice the first signs of symptomatic relief after some four to six weeks of taking the product regularly. There have, however, been many instances of people noting reactions within the first week of taking it and equally those of people who have gamely continued for six months before the first symptoms of relief became apparent. As with all medication a 'trial and error' process is involved.

In response to the second question the basic answer is no. Three distinct patterns of usage have developed with experience over the years. The first of the patterns is where the capsules have been taken regularly at the full dosage level until what are considered to be satisfactory results have been obtained. After this the product has not needed to be used again.

The second pattern has involved regular taking of the capsules until satisfactory results have been obtained, whereupon the dosage has been reduced to that of a daily maintenance course of one or two capsules only. In some cases this action has been found to be absolutely necessary to maintain a beneficial condition. If the capsules have been discontinued altogether the arthritic symptoms have recurred within two or three days in some instances. However, it must be pointed out that there are many cases where this pattern of usage is followed unnecessarily. Usually the explanation given by the person involved is that they are so afraid of a relapse that they prefer not to take any chances and do not mind taking a capsule or two each day as a maintenance course.

The third pattern has been that of taking the product at the full dosage until satisfactory results are obtained and then stopping completely. However, on a recurrence of symptoms, sometimes after several months, sometimes years, a short spell on the full dosage again has yielded another period of relief during which the capsules have not been necessary.

Will the Mussel Extract Prevent Arthritis?

Following on from these queries has been the question, 'Does the mussel extract have prophylactic properties?' In other words, if the product is taken on a regular basis by a person not suffering from arthritis, will it prevent that person from developing the disorder? The answer is that we do not know. There is no evidence at all to suggest that the product does have prophylactic properties and to obtain such evidence for a disorder of the nature of arthritis in general would be extremely difficult.

Non-specific Cases and Rheumatics in General

All the clinical trial work associated with the mussel extract has been related to diagnosed rheumatoid or osteo-arthritic cases. There have been, however, many reports of the use of the treatment in other forms of arthritis such as lumbago, bursitis, fibrositis or simply undiagnosed aches and pains. Whilst these particular conditions have not been subjected to specific clinical studies, there is sufficient evidence available, albeit subjective, from people in areas of the world ranging from tropical Africa through all the temperate zones to the Arctic regions of Scandinavia, Poland and Russia, to indicate that the symptoms of these can be alleviated by use of the product. This should not be surprising since the symptoms are basically similar to those of the two most common and serious forms of the disorder.

One of the more common expressions of how the mussel extract product has helped sufferers of non-specific, undiagnosed rheumatic conditions has been related to the people who find that they are a weather barometer. Such people are usually able to predict the onset of wet weather by their aching joints. After use of the extract they have claimed to be unable to do this since the aches have not appeared.

Other instances have simply related to the freedom from pain and stiffness during cold or damp weather. Nothing specific, nothing even definite except the better quality of life enjoyed through freedom from the usual, totally unspecific pains and aches.

Is it Harmful to Take More Than the Recommended Dose?

'Is the product dangerous or harmful if too much is taken?' This question has been asked many times and quite rightly too. It has been mentioned earlier in this book but is worthy of comment yet again that 'Natural' does not necessarily mean 'Safe'. Unfortunately the supposition that 'natural means safe' has too often been made by the natural health movement. That natural products are desirable is enthusiastically endorsed but caution must be exercised with regard to the selection and quantity of any substance consumed, be it natural or synthetic.

The mussel extract product is quite safe to use at many times the recommended dose. There have been reports from people who have found that they obtained either better or perhaps more rapid results by taking double this dose. Toxicity studies in the laboratory have indicated that no toxic effects were observable in the test subjects at 120 times the standard dose. Although there is no evidence yet available from controlled clinical studies to support the suggestion that higher doses will yield faster or better results, there is a distinct possibility that this could well be the case. The recommended dose of approximately 1g of the extract per day is quite a low dose rate for the product.

Reactions With Other Medication

Might the mussel extract react with other medication being taken at the same time? Well, yes of course it may. This will depend entirely upon the nature of the medication. The general answer to this question is that the extract does not react unfavourably with the medication normally used in the treatment of arthritic disorders or with pain-killing preparations. Bearing in mind the composition of the extract this is not surprising.

When preparations for other bodily disorders are involved it is advisable to seek the advice of one's doctor. In fact when any other medication is being used it is advisable to seek the doctor's advice. This is not simply to ascertain that there will not be any adverse interaction between the mussel extract and the other medication but also to establish that the doctor is not carefully monitoring the progress of some specific aspect of the medication which may be changed or negated by the taking of another product without his or her knowledge.

In all the years that the product has been in general use there have not been any recorded incidents of unfavourable interactions between the extract and other medications.

What Sort of Results Can be Expected?

The extremes of benefit that have been experienced after use of the mussel extract product, ignoring for the moment the completely negative results, have ranged from the simple case of the person with arthritis in the hands who can write, knit or open screw-top jars again after being unable to do so for years, to the person who has been bedridden or confined to a wheelchair with constant pain and depression who can once again live a normal life, go dancing, do gardening and swim. The majority of cases lie somewhere between these two extremes.

It would not be fair to present all the success factors associated with the product without also discussing the failures. It has already been pointed out that nothing is, or in fact is ever likely to be, one hundred per cent effective. There have been cases where people have been quite distressed after persevering through pain and immobility whilst taking the mussel extract product only to find that it has not helped them at all. In some cases their condition has even deteriorated because they have spent time taking a treatment which was, for them, ineffective. Such people have been even more distressed when they have used the product if they have seen the benefit that a friend or relative has obtained. The question that these people ask is of course 'Why not me?' The simple answer is that we do not know and one can only hope that there is some other relatively harmless product that will help them.

Returning to the successful cases which, in clinical trials conducted in Glasgow in 1980, were indicated as being approximately 60 per cent of rheumatoid arthritis sufferers and over 30 per cent osteo-arthritis sufferers, the various degrees of response to this treatment can be described as follows.

Usually the first signs of benefit have been signified by a slight decrease in pain, sometimes accompanied by an increase in freedom of movement of the affected part. Descriptions of these first signs have been given as, 'I found that I was sleeping right through the night again' (this usually being related by a person having osteo-arthritis in the hip), or, 'I noticed that I was able to walk to the corner shop and back without pain and without having to keep stopping to rest.' Naturally there have been many other descriptions too. In the case of many ladies it has been that they have been able to comb their hair or reach down their back to zip up a dress. To the person who has not suffered arthritic pains and limitations these first signs of improvement may seem very trivial. Be assured that they are not. They are major achievements which yield much encouragement when one has been unable to do such things for some time.

As the degree of benefit increases then pain becomes less intense and less frequent, possibly disappearing completely. If movement has been limited it too becomes easier and freer until, in many cases, normal limb movement is achieved.

Having said this it is necessary to point out that different degrees of response are achieved by different cases. Some have lost all pain but still have some difficulty with movement; others may move freely but have occasional twinges of pain and so on. It has been noted over years of experience with the product that some really severe cases of long duration have responded almost one hundred per cent and full relief of symptoms has been achieved. Conversely there have been mild cases for which the treatment has been used in the early stages with only moderate success.

It does appear, from general experience as well as from the clinical trial results, that the age of a person or the duration of the disorder do not have any significance with regard to the degree of success of the treatment. The author has personally witnessed successful results in the treatment of people in their late seventies and also in a child of less than two years of age. There have also been several reports of school-age children with Still's disease experiencing success with the mussel extract capsules.

Couldn't the Results be Psychological or Due to Natural Remission?
Yes, no doubt some of the successful results could be due to the powerful effect of a psychological stimulus. However, there is sufficient evidence available to allow this suggestion to be

discounted as being the real cause of success. The clinical and laboratory work rule out the possibility of psychological influence during the testing of a product. In the case of clinical trials involving human patients this response is called the 'placebo effect'. It is a common factor in all trials of new products stemming from the hope or belief of the patient that the new material will help them. Accordingly, half the trial patients are given a placebo (simply a sugar capsule or other harmless but non-effective treatment) and the other half the trial substance. The effect of the two substances can then be compared and placebo or psychological influence ruled out or minimized. This has been done for the mussel extract product. Additionally, whilst still considering human patients, it has been shown in previous clinical research that the psychological effect will only last for up to about six weeks in general with patients suffering from arthritis. There are so many people enjoying total symptomatic relief after using the extract many years ago that there can be no question of psychology being the cause of this benefit.

Apart from human patients, many animals have been successfully treated with the mussel extract preparation. Although dogs and cats will readily accept the product, others animals such as horses will not. For such animals the product has been disguised within their feed. The fact that animals suffering various forms of arthritic disorder have responded so well to the product would completely rule out the question of psychological response.

It is known that arthritis is a naturally remissive condition and there is every possibility that some of the successful cases being attributed to the mussel extract may well have been due to natural remission coinciding with the use of the treatment. There is no argument here; we simply do not know. However, it is pertinent to point out that exactly the same comment can be made in relation to any other therapy and, even more importantly, as far as the patient is concerned it doesn't matter as long as normal health has been restored.

Are There Any Side-effects?
It is difficult to imagine that there is any substance that does not

have 'side' effects. Even an inert substance can have a side-effect such as blocking a passageway or causing a growth to occur. The question really should be — what *are* the side-effects, because the problems caused relate to the nature of, and then the degree of, such effects.

What may be stated for the mussel extract preparation is that it does not have any serious adverse side-effects, in particular those which are so commonly associated with anti-arthritic drug therapy.

A very important qualification of the above statement needs to be made at this point. The mussel extract product has been shown to have only the mild side-effects indicated below provided that it has come from the genuine source. It has been reported that some more serious side-effects have been noted in people who used imitation products of unknown composition and which obviously had not been subjected to the quality control programme described earlier in this book.

For the approved mussel extract product the side-effects have been reported as follows:

1. A classical allergy reaction has been experienced by some people involving nausea, dizziness and sometimes a skin rash. This reaction has been typical of that caused by an allergy to anything and has disappeared quite rapidly upon ceasing intake of the product.
2. A considerable number of people using the product have reported a significant exacerbation of pain, sometimes in parts of their body not previously associated with arthritic problems and sometimes accompanied by a tingling sensation. At times the pain has been quite severe. However, these reactions have been of a temporary nature and have usually preceded very good results.
3. Reports of flatulence, diarrhoea and mild constipation have been received from a significant number of subjects.

A Beneficial Side-effect!
Side-effects do not always have to be unpleasant. On the basis that

the mussel extract preparation has its main value in its anti-inflammatory or anti-arthritic activity then the activity about to be described could be classed as a side-effect but certainly a beneficial one.

In almost all cases where the extract has been used, be it for human or animal treatment, it has been observed that the 'vitality' or 'well-being' of the subject has been significantly enhanced. There have been instances where a human subject has gained no benefit as far as relief of pain or increased mobility is concerned but has 'felt so much better in themselves'. The common expression by human subjects has been 'I feel so much better, I feel like getting out and doing things.' Naturally, if such subjects are also responding to the product in the relief of their arthritic symptoms, they would probably feel like this anyway. However, the comment has occurred too frequently and too universally to be a simple matter of coincidence. Similarly with animals, a new vibrance has been so easily detectable. Owners have reported that their elderly and normally tired and lethargic dog has suddenly changed to an enthusiastic animal meeting them at the door with the lead in its mouth ready to go out walking. There are several reports of old dogs (particularly Labradors and German Shepherds) which were about to be put down due to age and infirmity but which have had three or four years more of enjoyable life as a result of renewed vigour after taking the mussel extract preparation for hip dysplasia.

One of the doctors involved in a clinical trial using the extract with human subjects commented in the paper reporting the trial that one of the most difficult aspects of patient response to the mussel extract treatment to quantify was the feeling of 'well-being'.

It is the author's opinion that this factor may play a part in the general response of an arthritic patient to the treatment. There could be little doubt that if a patient began to feel better in themselves with a desire to be active, the response to the anti-arthritic treatment would be enhanced.

Use of the Preparation by Athletes

A natural follow-on from the section above has been the use of the mussel extract preparation by people involved in athletics or endurance sports. This activity has not come about through advertising of the product for this type of use but simply because experience of the people themselves has indicated a certain value in this respect.

There is no clinically proven evidence available to the author's knowledge to support the supposition that the mussel extract product aids athletic performance. In fact it is the opinion of the author that the product would not be capable of making, for example, a runner go faster than he or she was normally capable of doing. However, it is reasonable to speculate that if the product enhances the runner's vitality it may enhance endurance, thus allowing the person to run at maximum speed for a longer period. This is pure speculation but is an attempt to explain the fact that athletes in several different sports claim that use of the mussel extract has enhanced their performance.

A few years ago the British newspapers were carrying the story of a well-known athlete who had just won a major sporting event. The athlete claimed that he had only recently returned to the sport as a result of his recovery from a severe arthritic condition. He also claimed that his recovery was attributable to the mussel extract product which had been brought to his attention by a football trainer whose team were regular users.

Two further cases involve marathon runners, both New Zealanders. In one instance the subject is an elderly lady (in her 80s) who is still running, and winning, important veteran marathon events. The other concerns a middle-aged man who, having been forced to give up running through arthritis, felt so fit and well after using the mussel extract that he began marathon running again. He has since competed favourably in major international events in the USA, Europe and Japan.

Can This Property of the Mussel Extract be Explained?

There is no firm clinical evidence yet available to prove that the preparation is beneficial in the way that the athletes have described. Such evidence, when available, will possibly suggest the mechanism by which the extract creates the 'vitality' or 'feeling of well-being' factor associated with the product. However, considering certain known factors relating to the physiology of the human system and to the composition of the mussel extract preparation it is possible to speculate on a possible explanation.

It is known that stimulation of the adrenal gland to release the hormone cortisol can create a feeling of euphoria. Also, of course, release of the adrenocorticoids is known to influence carbohydrate and protein metabolism. It is natural to assume that these effects could lead to a desire to be active, and possibly also to enhanced physical endurance.

The mussel extract preparation contains an enzyme called sulphatase. Such enzymes have the ability to convert substances such as cortisol sulphate naturally present in the body into free cortisol. Although this specific reaction has not been established for the extract, part of the work with the mussel *Perna canaliculus* did demonstrate the ability to cleave the sulphate group from the sulphate conjugate. This work was done under laboratory conditions during a research programme and does not prove that the speculation made above is justified. It does, however, lend some support to the idea that it might be so.

Use of the Preparation With Animals

Animals also suffer arthritic complaints. In many cases it is almost inevitable that pet animals will develop forms of arthritis in their later years due to the unnatural lifestyle that they lead through being pets. In particular this applies to large dogs such as Alsatians, Labradors, Samoyed, Old English sheepdogs and such. Many of these dogs tend to be overweight and, for their size and build, under-exercised.

Horses used for racing which are regularly trained on hard ground or even sealed roads can develop joint problems in their legs. Whilst in some instances the cause of the problems suffered by the animals is not arthritic, the symptoms created by the problem are the same as those for arthritic disorders, i.e. swelling, pain and stiffness, and tend to respond to the same treatments, i.e. anti-inflammatory agents.

The mussel extract preparation (not in capsulated form but as tablets or, for horses, in powder form) has been used successfully with cats, dogs, horses and other animals. Naturally the main use has been with the three types just mentioned.

It has been noted that, in general, dogs and cats have responded to the treatment more quickly then human subjects. In most cases a positive response has been noticeable within seven to ten days of starting on the product.

The indications that an animal is responding to this treatment have almost always been described as a distinct change in attitude from lethargic to vibrant, brighter eyes, shiny, healthy coat and, frequently, in old dogs renewed puppy-like behaviour.

It is probably true to say that the most effective demonstration of the effectiveness of the mussel extract product which eliminates psychological, scientific and all other influences, is that of its use with arthritic dogs. The results are there to witness.

4

The Scientific Evaluation of New Zealand Green Mussel Extract

This chapter is included so that the results of laboratory and clinical research carried out on the New Zealand green mussel extract may be assessed. It is hoped that it will be of interest to non-technical readers despite the necessary use of some technical terminology.

Copies of all the papers or articles referred to in this resumé of research are available from either the author or McFarlane Laboratories NZ Ltd., PO Box 19028 Auckland, New Zealand.

The chapter follows chronologically the main individual studies conducted on the product, with personal commment on each. Much of the work reported in this chapter has been published in scientific journals as referenced.

Commencing in 1974 a number of studies have been conducted with the object of evaluating the efficacy of the mussel extract as a treatment for certain arthritic disorders. The studies have involved both human and animal trial subjects.

In 1974, a seven-week feed trial using rats was carried out in New Zealand at the Auckland School of Medicine[1]. The trial used twenty-eight adult albino rats equally divided between males and females with an induced experimental poly-arthritis. A modified Freunds adjuvant injected intradermally into the footpad of the rats created the poly-arthritis.

Fourteen of the rats were fed a diet of standard laboratory pellets. The other fourteen rats were fed a diet composed of the standard laboratory pellets to which powdered mussel extract had been added at the level of 1g of extract per kilogram of pellets.

Assessment of the arthritis score was graded according to the number of joints affected in each paw. The conclusion of this trial was that the mussel extract did not show any beneficial effect in the induced poly-arthritis in the rat.

It is worth noting that there were shortcomings in this study which make the drawing of any firm conclusions open to question. One criticism is that there is no indication of the amount of trial preparation consumed by individual animals. Thus no figures for rate of dosage per kilogram body weight are available. Also the amount of mussel extract added to the pellets (1g per kg) is rather light for a study of this type.

In a volume of the *New Zealand Medical Journal* the results of a 'Pilot Study on the Effect of New Zealand Green Mussel on Rheumatoid Arthritis'[2] were published. The trial was conducted in 1974 at the University of Otago Medical School, in Dunedin, New Zealand.

Six patients with symptoms which were considered to be potentially reversible by therapy and who had had rheumatoid arthritis for periods ranging from two months to twenty years were involved in a double-blind crossover trial. The period of allocation of randomized 'active' or placebo capsules was twelve weeks, six weeks on each course. Patients other than those on maintenance gold or low-dose steroid therapy were taken off all but analgesic drugs for a period of fourteen days prior to the trial. Assessments of patient response were made at regular intervals throughout the trial and involved measurements of, and questions for, the standard parameters. Five patients completed this trial. One (who had received only a placebo) was unable to continue due to a deterioration in condition.

The study conclusion indicated that the mussel extract did not show any greater effect than a placebo in a double-blind crossover trial on five people.

The main criticism of this study must be that the number of patients involved was too small to allow any conclusion to be drawn at all. It is also important to recognize that a standard and short-term crossover trial is not suitable for evaluating the therapeutic efficacy of a preparation which is slow-acting but has relatively long-term effects. In support of this statement it is only necessary to consider the 'carry-over' effect which would be experienced by a patient receiving the active preparation first. If a preparation giving relatively long-term relief of symptoms is involved under these conditions then screening of any placebo effect could be expected. To allow an adequate 'wash-out' period at the crossover may cause unnecessary suffering and possibly further deterioration in the condition of those patients who had received the placebo first.

Finally, whilst collectively the results of the five patients show no significant improvement due to the use of the mussel extract, a study of the individual results does suggest that one or two out of the five patients were showing improvement. However, the conclusions of this trial are invalid due to the small number of patients.

Between 1974 and 1976 several investigative projects involving the mussel extract were undertaken by research centres with an interest in marine pharmacology. Thus studies (*in vitro*) carried out at the Shizuoka College of Pharmacy in Japan[3] indicated that fractions of the extract demonstrated antihistamine and adenosine triphosphate promoting activity.

Also antihistamine and anti-oedemic activity was reported following studies carried out on mouse and rat models at private research centres in Japan and Australia.[4]

A study conducted in Switzerland in 1976 using female rat models with adjuvant-induced arthritis[5] noted that an anti-inflammatory activity of the mussel extract could be observed in the non-injected foot whereas the swelling in the injected foot was not influenced. This led the report to conclude with the observation that the inhibitory effect of the extract on the secondary lesions seemed to be an immunological effect.

An interesting aspect of this particular study is that the mussel extract preparation was administered orally. Up to this point only intra-peritoneal administration of the material had indicated any anti-inflammatory activity, all oral administration having failed to indicate a response.

Also in 1976 a preliminary clinical trial involving human subjects was commenced at the Homoeopathic Hospital in Glasgow, Scotland.[6] This trial involved 56 patients, 46 of whom were suffering from rheumatoid arthritis and 10 from osteo-arthritis. All the patients were chronic cases and had failed to respond to orthodox or homoeopathic treatment.

The patients were all maintained on their existing therapy and mussel extract was given additionally at a dosage of 3×350mg capsules per patient per day. As the patients were not improving on the existing therapy it was considered that improvements which took place were due to the addition of the extract to the treatment regime. No placebo patients were involved in the trial.

Assessments of patient response were made at the start of the trial, then at fortnightly intervals for six weeks and then monthly. The trial did not run for a fixed term but continued for over three years with the minimum term being three months. Assessment parameters were those normally associated with trials involving arthritic patients.

As this study was considered to be of a preliminary nature only, with the aim of indicating the need, and suitable design protocol, for a more defined trial, the results were not published. They indicated, however, that approximately 60 per cent of the patients with rheumatoid arthritis and 30 per cent of those with osteo-arthritis benefited from the addition of the mussel extract to their treatment. It was also pointed out in the trial report that, of the rheumatoid patients who benefited, approximately half improved considerably and half improved only moderately. With reference to the osteo patients the report advises that only those patients with generalized osteo-arthritis improved. The patients with single joint osteo-arthritis showed no benefit.

No significant changes were noted in blood counts, serum biochemistry or serology in the trial patients as a whole. However, in one patient the R3 value changed from positive to negative and in a few cases the haemoglobin values improved.

This preliminary study led to a six-month double-blind trial being conducted at the Victoria Infirmary and the Homoeopathic Hospital in Glasgow during 1980.[7] In the double-blind study, 60 patients were on the waiting list of the Victoria Infirmary for orthopaedic surgery. Of these, 28 of the patients suffered from clinical rheumatoid arthritis and 38 had clinical and radiological evidence of osteo-arthritis.

The patients were asked to continue all previous therapy unchanged, the mussel extract or placebo capsules being additional to their regular treatment. For the first three months of the trial period the patients were treated with randomly allocated double-blind therapy. For the second three months all patients were treated with the 'active' preparation. Full assessment took place at the three-month and six-month terms in addition to routine monthly assessments throughout.

The results of this six-month double-blind study were similar to those of the longer-term preliminary study in that 67.9 per cent of the rheumatoid patients and 39.5 per cent of the osteo patients were reported to have benefited from the mussel extract treatment.

An interesting aspect which was reported in the discussion section of the published results of this study relates to the comparison of the extract with gold and Levamisole therapy. The observation is made that the mussel extract was as effective as gold though not as effective as Levamisole in improving pain, stiffness and grip strength. However gold and Levamisole are both second-line treatments with a relatively high incidence of toxic side-effects. Table 3, reproduced with the kind permission of *The Practitioner*, compares

Table 3. Comparison of drop-out and side-effect rates on treatment with *Perna canaliculus* (present trial), and gold and levamisole (El-Ghobary *et. al.*, 1978)

	Perna canaliculus	Treatment Gold	Levamisole
Drop-out rate	12%	55%	60%
Side-effect rate	13.6%	35%	45%

the side-effects and patient drop-out rates of the three preparations. In 1980 Rainsford and Whitehouse published a paper relating to a gastro-protective property discovered in mussel extract.[8] At the University of Tasmania Medical School, Hobart and the John Curtin School for Medical Research, Canberra, Australia, preliminary studies to assess the therapeutic benefits of oral treatment of rats with combined preparations of the mussel extract preparation and acetylsalicylic acid were carried out. These studies indicated that rats given a mixture of the mussel extract preparation and acetylsalicylic acid developed much less gastric mucosal damage than rats given acetylsalicylic acid alone. This observation led to the study of the gastro-protective plus anti-inflammatory properties of the mussel extract preparation so reported.

Cold-stressed male and female Wistar Hooded rat models were used in the evaluation of the combined anti-inflammatory and gastro-protective properties of the crude extract and lipid fractions of the extract in admixture with non-steroidal anti-inflammatory drugs of known ulcerogenic character. Anti-inflammatory response was measured using the carrageenan-induced rat footpad oedema. Gastro-protectivity was determined by visual observation of the number and severity of lesions in the gastric mucosa.

Long-term studies related to the gastro-protective effect were carried out using female, Landrace X Large White Cross strain pigs with oral dosing of NSAI drug/crude extract or NSAI drug/lipid fraction mixtures. Gastro-protective effectiveness was determined by postmortem observation of the number and severity of macroscopic lesions in the gastric and upper intestinal mucosa.

The results of these studies are of considerable interest since they indicate that the anti-inflammatory property of the mussel extract acted synergistically with that of some of the NSAI drugs administered concomitantly. Additionally, and unlike many potential gastro-protectants, the mussel extract does not impair the therapeutic activity of low doses of the NSAI drugs but in fact enhances it.

The relative specificity of the extract from *Perna canaliculus* for these activities was demonstrated by comparison with similar extracts prepared from the blue mussel (*Mytilus edulis aoteanus*), the oyster (*Crassostrea glomerata*), the scallop (*Pecten novaezealandiae*) and the paua (abalone) (*Haliotis iris*). These other molluscs did not have the properties indicated by *Perna canaliculus*.

The gastro-protective activity associated with the lipid fractions of the mussel extract varied in function according to which NSAI drug was used. Thus the protective effects against indomethacin-induced gastric mucosal damage were predominant in the chloroform solvent aliquots after silicic chromatography of the crude lipid extract. The effects against aspirin-induced gastric mucosal damage, however, were predominant in those lipids present in the acetone and methanol fractions after silicic acid chromatography.

The results of this work also suggested that the activity of the mussel extract preparation in minimizing gastric damage caused by NSAI drugs is unique and is not due to the presence of a crude bulk substance.

A study published in the *New Zealand Medical Journal* in September 1980 gave the results of carefully controlled experiments in which the anti-inflammatory activity of mussel extract was determined using animal models.[9] These experiments involved the use of male and female Dark Agouti rats with administration of the mussel extract by the oral route, gastric gavage and intra-peritoneal injection.

Anti-inflammatory response was measured by the reduction in carrageenan-induced inflammatory oedema of the rat footpad resulting from administration of the mussel preparation. The response was compared with that produced by administration of a proven anti-inflammatory drug (aspirin). The administrators were well aware of the limitations of methods involving the use of intra-peritoneal administration of test substances and were careful to demonstrate the specificity of the injected material.

The results of this study indicated that the crude extract of the mussel (*Perna canaliculus*) exhibits a marked anti-inflammatory effect when administered by the intra-peritoneal route. The effect was specific and was also shown to be cumulative. Administration of the preparation by the oral route, however, did not initiate anti-inflammatory response.

The *British Medical Journal* of 25 April 1981 carried a 'short report' with the heading 'Seatone is ineffective in rheumatoid arthritis'. This report was the result of a short crossover trial conducted at St Bartholomew's Hospital, London,[10] in which thirty patients with rheumatoid arthritis took part. It involved treatment with the mussel extract for four weeks and treatment with a placebo for four weeks. All the patients were on treatment which was not adequately controlling their condition and they remained on this treatment throughout the trial. Four patients did not complete the trial, three due to minor side-effects and one for reasons not related to the trial. The standard parameters related to arthritic trial patients were assessed at the beginning and end of the study and at the end of each treatment period.

The trial concluded that no significant difference had been demonstrated between the extract and placebo treatments. It was also reported that a very considerable placebo effect was evident and that it was not surprising that several patients responded well.

Two observations relating to the reporting of this study are immediately evident. First it is not possible to claim that the mussel extract is ineffective using the results of a small, short-term trial such as this. Second, the fact that the trial involved a crossover coupled with the short term made it unsuitable for evaluating a product of this type.

The table of measurements presented in the report of the study and reproduced as Table 4 shows a definite trend towards improvement in patients being treated. Whilst it cannot be said with certainty, it is likely that an extended time period for this trial would have produced a different conclusion. For instance, with a longer-term study it is most unlikely that a placebo response would have persisted and the mussel-extract-treated patients would have had a chance to respond fully.

One further comment is that a high placebo response was to

be expected in this particular trial due to the fact that all the patients actually requested the mussel extract.

Some criticism of the Glasgow double-blind study which was contained in the report of this trial has been fully answered in a letter to the *British Medical Journal*.[20]

Table 4.   Means of measurements made at start of study and at end of each treatment period.

	Pain score	Duration of morning stiffness (mins.)	Articular index	Proximal inter-phalangeal joint size (mm)	Analgesic consumption (number of tablets)
Initially	12.3	43.7	11.5	567.7	
After Seatone	11.0	30.6	9.0	569.3	58.8
After placebo	11.5	34.2	9.0	568.8	66.5

Also in 1981 the results of long-term toxicity and teratological trials conducted in the Department of Medicine University of Auckland became available.[12,13] These results indicated that the product, even at high doses had no toxic or adverse teratological effect. The objective of the toxicological testing was to determine the effect of the mussel extract on biological processes and to obtain data on the characteristics of the product related to dosage and toxicity.

The study was carried out in two phases. In one the response of both male and female rats to a single high dose of product was determined. In the second phase the effect of repeated administration of high doses was analysed. The purpose of the first phase was to determine the LD 50 for the product and the very high dose of 8g/kg was used. The purpose of the second phase was to extend the information to cover a longer term of administration. In this case the animals were fed at the rate of 2g/kg continuously for fourteen days.

The results of these tests indicated that at the dose level of 8g/kg/day (equivalent to a dose of 560g in a person of 70kg body-weight) the product was not toxic. In fact it was not possible to determine a value for the LD 50 due to the absence of toxicity at such high doses. Further, the regular consumption of a high dose over a period of fourteen consecutive days did not produce any toxic effects.

The teratogenic study covering a period of five consecutive months was designed to assess the potential of the mussel extract product to influence foetal development during gestation in pregnant females taking the product on a regular basis. Studies were carried out using the progeny of two groups of rats. A control group was fed a standard diet and the other was fed the standard diet containing mussel extract at 54 times the recommended dose. Studies of the effect of the extract on the reproductive system were carried out using twenty breeding pairs each of a control and test group, which were fed either the standard diet or the diet containing mussel extract for ninety days prior to mating. Gonadal function, oestrus cycles, mating behaviour, conception rates, parturition, lactation and early development were then studied.

The results of the tests indicated that no teratogenic effects were observed at the doses used (54 times normal). Two differences between the control group and the mussel extract fed group were noted, however. These were that conception was delayed in the test animals (though equally the gestation period may have been prolonged), and the litter sizes born to the test animals were smaller than those born to the control group. However, the average weight of the progeny born to the test animals at both 4 and 21 days after birth was greater than that of the progeny born to the control group. It could be that the smaller litter size of the test animals contributed to this difference.

A pilot trial was conducted with greyhound dogs as the trial subjects. The aim of this study was to assess the suitability of the greyhound as a biological assay model in the evaluation of the mussel extract for anti-arthritic activity. The greyhound was selected as a possible model for several main reasons:

1. This animal is a 'commercial' species, thus early detection of disability due to arthritis is likely.
2. The animal is familiar with regular handling and examination.
3. The animal is used to a strict dietary and exercise programme.
4. Confinement to a kennel with only routine exercise is well tolerated.

During the seven-week period of the study the animals were all fed the same diet (the amount of food being related to body-weight), were subjected to the same handling and exercise and were housed in identical kennels all in the same area. The trial was of the double-blind design involving twelve dogs of which six received the mussel extract preparation and six received placebo. The mussel extract preparation was administered orally in capsulated form at the rate of 3×350mg capsules per dog per day. Placebo capsules identical in appearance and odour were similarly administered.

The results of this study indicated that the greyhound is not a suitable animal for this type of assay. This was due primarily to the difficulty experienced in measuring parameters which specifically indicated a change in the arthritic condition of the dogs. However, this trial, in conjunction with an additional uncontrolled study conducted during the same period as the trial but also continued for a much longer period, has provided some interesting and useful results.

The additional study involved six dogs. Three of these were taken from the group of six that had received the 'active' preparation in the trial. These three dogs has shown a marked improvement in condition, freedom of movement and pain. Two dogs were not involved in the trial but were suffering from an arthritic disorder which prevented them from exercising or racing. The sixth dog was a trial subject which had been on placebo and had shown a minor response. The four dogs from the trial were, at the end of the trial period treated at a higher dose (5×350mg capsules per day) of the mussel preparation. The other two dogs received the 5×350mg

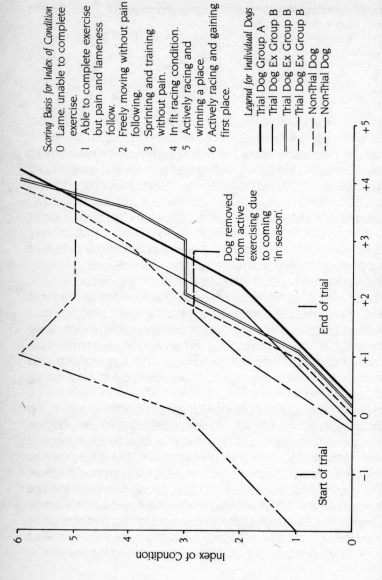

Scoring Basis for Index of Condition

0 Lame, unable to complete exercise.
1 Able to complete exercise but pain and lameness follow.
2 Freely moving without pain following.
3 Sprinting and training without pain.
4 In fit racing condition.
5 Actively racing and winning a place.
6 Actively racing and gaining first place.

Legend for Individual Dogs

Trial Dog Group A
Trial Dog Ex Group B
Trial Dog Ex Group B
Trial Dog Ex Group B
Non-Trial Dog
Non-Trial Dog

Dog removed from active exercising due to coming 'in season'.

End of trial

Start of trial

Index of Condition

Figure 5. Graph showing the change in condition of individual greyhound dogs which have been treated with Seatone

capsules per day dose throughout, one for a period of sixteen weeks and one for twenty-six weeks.

The improvement in the condition of these animals is clearly indicated in Fig. 5. Although the dogs became free-running, keen to work and free from pain, it is important to stress that, to date, this has not been objectively proven to be the result of a change in their arthritic disability.

In Australia at the Royal Melbourne Institute of Technology, some preliminary laboratory investigations were conducted during 1981.[11] The work involved a biochemical and pharmacological study of the mussel extract. The extract, supplied direct from New Zealand, was separated into three fractions representing the water-soluble phase, the lipid, i.e. fatty, phase and the residue.

In order to test the activity of the fractions a modified carrageenan-induced oedema assay was used in which two paws of the rat were challenged and monitored for volume changes over a period of hours. The challenges involved the extract, the various fractions, known anti-inflammatory drugs and controls (saline).

A departure from the conventional intra-peritoneal injection method of administration of test substances was introduced into this investigation. Using solubilization with pH adjustment and also liposomal carriers it was found that standardization of the mode of administration of the various samples, i.e. drugs, extracts and control was achieved. This was considered to be an improvement on the method in which one substance is introduced by intra-peritoneal injection and another by gastric gavage.

The conclusion from this work was that the mussel extract possessed significant anti-inflammatory activity which appeared to be associated with the non-lipid fractions. The inference was therefore that the active material is water-soluble and polar in nature.

Concurrently in the Department of Medicine, University of Auckland, a Research Fellowship was sponsored by McFarlane Laboratories Ltd to investigate the pharmacology and chemistry of the New Zealand mussel extract.[14] This study involved a detailed investigation into the fractionation of the mussel extract and the possible modes of action by which the anti-inflammatory activity might function.

Experiments to ascertain whether the extract behaved as a first- or second-line treatment were conducted as were specificity studies to establish that the activity was limited to the mussel *Perna canaliculus*. For this second part of the study shellfish from the same area of the sea in which the green mussel samples were cultivated were used.

A secondary study by another research group had already investigated the influence of geographical location within the species of *Perna canaliculus* itself. The conclusion of this work was that the activity was specific to *Perna canaliculus* and that it was probably associated with a high molecular weight protein compound.

Further work in the Department of Medicine at Auckland University, subsequently published in the *New Zealand Medical Journal*, supported these observations and found that the anti-inflammatory activity of the extract could be isolated in a fraction representing only 16 per cent by weight of the parent extract. [15]

One aspect of the laboratory work which attracted a good deal of criticism was that little or no evidence of efficacy had been demonstrated by oral administration of the mussel extract. This aspect was addressed by Dr T. E. Miller and Dr H. Wu at the University of Auckland in a novel experiment. [16]

It was known that prostaglandin synthetase inhibitors such as aspirin, naprosen and indomethacin interfere with ovulation and prolong the gestation period in the rat. A trial was conducted in which rats were fed the mussel extract preparation and the effects on parturition and foetal development were observed. The observations made as a result of this work were consistent with the known effects of non-steroidal anti-inflammatory drugs. This suggested that the mussel extract does contain pharmacologically active material which inhibits prostaglandin biosynthesis. Further, it is established that this effect of the extract could be demonstrated using the oral route of administration.

In 1983 the results of a short-term trial carried out at Auckland Hospital were published in the *New Zealand Medical Journal*.[17] This trial involved forty-seven outpatients with active classical or definite rheumatoid arthritis. The patients were selected such that none of the trial subjects had been taking steroids, gold, chloroquine or d-penicillamine.

For the first six weeks of the trial the patients were treated with a proven anti-inflammatory drug (naproxen) plus the mussel extract, the other half receiving naproxen plus a placebo. For the second six-week period the naproxen was replaced by a placebo for both groups of patients. The standard assessments for changes in arthritic condition were applied to all patients during the period of the trial. Patient compliance, as evidenced by drop-out rate, was used as the method of assessing the effectiveness of the treatments.

The conclusion of the trialists was that the similar drop-out rate in both groups of patients undergoing the trial demonstrated that neither placebo nor mussel extract alone provided adequate relief of symptoms in the majority of patients despite six weeks previous treatment. It was acknowledged that Gibson and others have suggested that the mussel extract may have an effect which becomes apparent only after three to six months, but it was not possible to confirm this factor in this particular trial.

In commenting on the conclusions from this trial it is fair to point out that the drop-out rate of patients can, unfortunately, often be due to factors not connected directly with the treatment. For instance, patients can become irritated with perhaps long periods of waiting at the outpatients clinic, particularly if infrequent bus services or long journeys are also involved.

Another comment would be that it is unfortunate that this trial could not have proceeded for a longer period as, although it is recognized that there was a high drop-out rate in both trial groups immediately naproxen was withdrawn, the number of patients receiving the mussel extract who remained in the trial was double that of those who were receiving a placebo.

Finally, it is fair to comment that naproxen is a potent and fast-acting drug and the sudden withdrawal of such a preparation from the patients would be quite likely to produce the effects shown in the trial even against other 'proven' but perhaps slow-acting drug products.

A six-month, placebo-controlled study at the Centre for Rheumatic Diseases, Glasgow suggested that Seatone was not effective in rheumatoid arthritis.[18]

This trial involved thirty-five patients with diagnosed rheumatoid arthritis which was not being adequately controlled by non-steroidal anti-inflammatory drugs. The patients continued to take their regular drug therapy and mussel extract or placebo capsules were given additionally.

The standard assessments used in studies to determine the effectiveness of anti-arthritic preparations were made at the beginning, middle and end of the trial period.

It must be pointed out that this trial was judging the mussel extract on the basis of its ability to improve the condition of patients who were already not adequately helped by powerful drugs, (one patient was on prednisolone). Further, only twenty patients received the mussel extract, the other fifteen received a placebo.

On the basis of only twenty people, who were already regarded as difficult to treat with conventional therapy, it is not considered fair to conclude that the mussel extract is of no benefit in arthritis. The mussel extract has, in fact, been very effective in some cases of rheumatoid arthritis that had not responded to a wide range of drug therapy. However, it could not be expected that this would always be the case.

Japanese researchers have been interested in New Zealand green mussel extract since it first became commercially available in 1974. At the University of Shizuoka near Tokyo, studies were undertaken by Professor T. Kosuge to investigate the anti-arthritic activity of the mussel extract from a different angle altogether to the conventional Western one. Professor Kosuge had been involved for some time in an investigation of the preparations used in Chinese Medicine in an effort to determine and isolate the pharmacologically active principles of these compounds. He decided to approach the activity of the mussel extract preparation in a similar manner.

The main work done at Shizuoka involved observations on the effect of the extract on blood cells, and haemostatic defence systems plus some investigation into possible enzyme-promoting activity in ADP-ATP reactions. Although Professor Kosuge's speciality is the isolation and characterization of pharmacologically active components in natural substances, he suggested that experimentation using the whole extract rather than a specific isolate of the extract was appropriate. This reasoning fitted into the philosophy of Chinese medication principles. However, it was also the opinion of Professor Kosuge that the active principle in the extract could be highly unstable and thus, not only very difficult to isolate for identification but also ineffective once isolated from the parent extract.

The demonstration by the Shizuoka University workers of the significant and measurable effect of the mussel extract on blood activity was able to be correlated with the anti-inflammatory activity as determined using the carrageenan-induced oedema assay. This was valuable and significant evidence in that it suggests that the measurements made by the Shizuoka researchers, based on the Chinese Medicine approach were directly related to anti-inflammatory measurements as determined by a standard, Western medicine method. Thus it was possible that the haemostatic defence measurements were directly related to anti-inflammatory activity.

During the last part of 1984 and the greater part of 1985 clinical trials were carried out in France.[19] The trials involved two institutions, Lariboisière and Pitié Saltpétrie hospitals. One of the hospitals investigated the use of the mussel extract in osteo-arthritis and the other studied its use in rheumatoid arthritis.

The two trials were double-blind, placebo-controlled, involving a total of 120 patients for a term of six months. Also, very careful matching of patients involved in the trials was enforced. This prolonged the overall period of the trials but was considered worthwhile.

The trials were in the charge of Professors Audeval and Bouchacourt and were conducted strictly according to the protocol detailed in the *European Directive on Clinical Trials of New Drugs Against Rheumatism*.

Whilst, at the time of writing, the details of these studies have not yet been published, it has been reported that statistically significant results indicating that the mussel extract is beneficial in the treatment of arthritic disorders were obtained.

Finally, a new clinical study of a different nature is currently underway in France. This study is in the form of a double-blind, placebo-controlled, clinical trial involving one hundred patients undergoing radiation therapy in the treatment of cancer.

This work has come about as a result of a most interesting observation that some arthritic patients using the mussel extract who, coincidentally, were receiving radiation treatment, did not develop the inflammatory condition associated with radiation treatment.

A preliminary, uncontrolled trial with forty-three patients confirmed that the extract did appear to prevent the onset of inflammation.

As the inflammatory condition induced by radiation therapy is a very painful one, and can, in fact, limit the amount of radiation treatment that can be given, the possibility of a simple and safe preventative therapy being available is of considerable importance.

The results of the double-blind trial presently underway when statistically analysed will indicate whether or not this prophylactic effect of the mussel extract can be scientifically proven.

Summary
Table 5 presents an abbreviated summary of the results of trials carried out on New Zealand green mussel extract to date. As no other trial work or studies have been reported or published it is assumed that this is the total information available on this subject at the present time.

Table 5. A Summary of the Evaluation Studies Conducted on New Zealand Mussel Extract (Seatone)

Year	Location	Nature of Study	Subject Model	Result
1974	New Zealand: Auckland Medical School	Adjuvant-induced polyarthritis (published)	Rats	No effect demonstrated
1974	New Zealand: Otago Medical School	Double-blind crossover trial (12 weeks) (published)	Humans (R.A.) (6)	No effect demonstrated
1976	Japan: Shizuoka College of Pharmacy	Antihistamine and ATP-ase promoting activity	(In vitro) Guinea pig ileum	Positive effects demonstrated
1976	Japan/Australia: Private Research Institute	Antihistamine and anti-oedemic activity	Rats	Positive effects demonstrated
1976	Switzerland: Private Research Institute	Adjuvant-induced arthritis	Rats	Positive effects demonstrated
1976-80	United Kingdom: Glasgow Homoeopathic Hospital	Controlled clinical study (preliminary) (3 months-3 years)	Humans (R.A. & OA) (56)	Positive effects demonstrated

Year	Institution	Study	Subject	Result
1979	Australia: University of Tasmania Medical School and National University of Australia John Curtin Med. Res. School	Gastro-protective and Anti-inflammatory activity (published)	White Cross Pigs	Positive effects demonstrated
1980	United Kingdom: Victoria Infirmary and Homoeopathic Hospitals Glasgow	Controlled double-blind clinical trial (published)	Humans (RA. & OA) (66)	Positive effects
1981	New Zealand: Contracted Research	Toxicity evaluations	Rats	Not toxic
1981	New Zealand: Contracted Research	Teratogenic evaluation	Rats	Not teratogenic
1980-1	Auckland University	Lab studies to demonstrate anti-inflammatory activity (published)	Rats	Positive effects demonstrated
1981	United Kingdom: St Bartholomew's Hospital	Controlled clinical crossover trial (8 wks) (published)	Humans (RA.) (30)	No effect demonstrated
1980 (contin.)	Royal Melbourne Institute of Technology	Fractionation studies combined with bio-assays for active principle identification	Rats	Positive results

1983-4	Auckland University	Lab studies to investigate pharmacological mechanisms of extract (published)	Rats	Positive results
1981-2	Auckland University	Fractionation of extract to find active principle (published)	Rats	Positive results
1984	Auckland University	Demonstration of prostaglandin inhibitory activity (published)	Rats	Positive results
1981	New Zealand: Auckland Hospital	Controlled clinical trial (12 wks) (published)	Humans (R.A.) (47)	No effect demonstrated
1983	Centre for Rheumatic Diseases Glasgow	Six month trial on 35 patients	Humans (35)	No effect demonstrated
1984-5	France: Paris	Six month double-blind clinical evaluations, on specific arthritic patients (to be published)	Humans (120) (R.A. & O.A.)	Positive activity
Contin. (1974) on	Japan: Shizuoka College	Activity measurement and stability factor studies	Mice and rats	Positive activity

5

The Results: What Users Say

Critics may say that the inclusion of the personal experiences in this chapter is characteristic of quackery. They will point out that the personal experiences of people suffering or being treated for disorders are too subjective for them to have value in assessment of the results of the treatment, and that only strictly objective assessments, devoid of any emotional content can accurately assess the progress of the disease or its treatment.

All of this criticism is, in fact, true, but it is only true under certain circumstances. It is the author's considered opinion that

1. the statements above represent an extremist view which, in itself, is an emotive one, and
2. there is really no such thing as a totally 'objective' assessment, particularly of the arthritic diseases.

In almost all instances, certainly in trials of anti-arthritic drugs, a considerable part of the assessment involves a question-and-answer programme in which the patient gives details of pain, duration of morning stiffness and such parameters. These are subjective evaluations and are just the same as those given by letter or telephone and upon which this chapter is based.

If the experiences are genuine, are sufficient in number and diversity of origin, and cover a reasonable duration of time, then there can be absolutely no question of quackery being involved. In fact such experiences represent a very valuable source of medical information which in some instances is more relevant than that which could be gained in a short-term clinical trial.

The experiences which are quoted in this chapter come from people in countries spanning the whole world. Some of the writers have themselves been medical doctors and specialists and the letters have covered a period of ten years. In some cases the original communication advising of success with the product has been followed up years later with further communications confirming that the results were still as good. In most cases the patient involved has had his or her condition correctly diagnosed by the doctor. It is not simply a matter of non-specific cases responding to the treatment.

Why do People Bother to Write at all?

There are several different reasons for the letters and telephone calls commenting on the results of treatment with the mussel extract product. In many cases the communication has been a comment on results followed by a query such as, 'Is it necessary to continue taking the capsules indefinitely?' or, perhaps, 'What level of maintenance dose is recommended?' In others the comment on results has been followed by a query about supplies to a friend or relative in another country.

Another type of communication has explained in detail the results of the treatment with mussel extract. This detail has been given because the person concerned has been so grateful after having had most of the conventional drug therapy without success, thus feeling that there was little hope for recovery. In some instances the communications from medical specialists have also been quite detailed as such people are used to recording and noting details of disease or treatment prognosis.

Some communications are just expressions of gratitude from people who are relieved to have found something which has helped them. Naturally such communications would be received by anyone who had supplied something which helped a person to recover from a crippling and painful disease. However, in the case of the hundreds of such letters or telephone calls received about the mussel extract treatment, much valuable information about the disease state, the time before results appeared, duration of relief, etc., has been gained. It should be remembered that these communications are unsolicited, natural responses from people who have purchased a product. They are not the response of test groups which have been given free samples.

Why Include these Details in the Book?

No apology is made for including comments and excerpts from the communications referred to. The comfort that so many people feel, through hearing what someone else with almost identical symptoms or case history to theirs has to say about a treatment, makes it worthy of inclusion. All the quotations used are absolutely genuine and are the true sentiments of people who have felt so relieved or pleased that they wanted to advise the manufacturing company or the author personally of their success. Some of the excerpts which follow relate to humans and some to animals. Obviously only a few examples can be included here but it is hoped that they will indicate that the patient's 'subjective' views do in fact represent an expert opinion, that of the sufferer!

The letters quoted here cover the period 1975 to 1985. The names of the writers have been omitted to save them any possible embarrassment. Also the name of the product has had to be omitted to be consistent with the rest of the book.

An example of the amount of detail which some of the reports have included is given in the following two excerpts from a letter received from England and another from Spain.

Further to our telephone conversation in May last, I can now advise you further of my progress with a little more confidence than I had at that time. You will recall that I was suffering a 'flare-up' and although it was a nuisance I know enough now not to get too despondent.

I therefore continued with five capsules per day and gritted my teeth! From a purely clinical approach I think the best I can do is itemize the pattern of things as they stand at present.

1. The latest flare-up from inception to completion has lasted approximately two months. It commenced noticeably about the beginning of May last. I had unusual stress at the time with family problems too.

2. Since roughly a week ago (3rd July) the pain has dramatically eased. At first I thought it was wishful thinking and could not have abated. (I always think this when it seems too good to be true!). However, I have now been moving around with greater comfort continually for a week and therefore feel confident to announce publicly that I have reached another stage of healing.

3. Once again my leg has the sensation of being longer — although I realize it is obviously the muscles getting stronger and therefore regaining their natural shape and size after their wastage.

4. Because the leg appears more elastic I do not have the terrible pulling and burning pain in my right buttock, back and indeed the whole of the trunk of my body. I appeared at one time to have lost the whole muscle power four-dimensional, i.e. length, front, back and side!

Measured against the state I was in a year ago, it is a joy not to continually tremble, especially in the trunk of my body — absolutely no control over the nerves it would seem at the time. So — from this standpoint — a very great measure of improvement in strength.

5. Still a marked presence of ammonia in body wastage, especially at the end of the day.

6. When I stand I am able to have both knees nearly level as opposed to having to bend the 'good' leg to accommodate the affected leg approximately 5″. I am able to walk in the fashion of heel-toe now without distress, instead of walking

on my toes on that foot because the back of the leg just could not stretch down. The whole leg appears more flexible.

7. My conclusion is that when I suffer pain, it is a good sign because when it clears my leg has certainly been getting back to normal in all ways. The calf muscles have regained their proper shape and it is not so obvious that they are wasted when measured against the good leg.

8. I am able to walk a short way indoors without the aid of a walking stick and without falling heavily over to one side each time I place my foot to the ground. The footsteps I have been taking in the last couple of days have been normally balanced and most important of all, there has been no pain, not even a feeling of soreness in the joints when I have placed my foot to the ground.

9. I do not intend to try walking outdoors without the aid of the walking stick until nature shows me without doubt that all is back to normal. I intend to continue to take 5 capsules a day until I am walking without the stick and still without pain — perhaps to the extent of taking a whole bottleful before the next step. I then propose to drop my daily intake to four capsules per day for maybe a full bottle, then three capsules for a full bottle.

I think that if I can get to the happy stage of no pain and back to normal I shall, for as long as the extract is produced continue to take one capsule a day for the rest of my life.

10. The whole limb appears to have been lubricated because I cannot remember now the sickening noise resembling castanets or dry twigs breaking when I endeavoured to bend the limb. I have been taking the (mussel extract) at full prescribed dosage continually since the commencement of last August, therefore it is the best part of a year now, and when deliberately comparing my strength to this time last year it is astonishing how near I am to being normal again!

Another example of the type of detailed letter received is from a gentleman in Spain.

To conclude this year I feel obliged to inform you about my miraculous experience with (the mussel extract). I already told you something of my background in my first letter and that I badly suffered with rheumatoid poly-arthritis during the past months. From August on I have been treated here with all hard medical drugs of the pirarolones, butaphenarolone and corticosteroid groups without any lasting results. Sometimes a certain relief but upon ceasing with a specific medication after a few days from bad to worse again. My whole condition became gradually worse. I felt poisoned by medicines, lost my appetite and felt depressed. No wonder as I saw the wheelchair coming towards me. I stopped therefore all cures and felt a little better when the side-effects disappeared. At that time the balance was: active arthritis in the right knee accompanied by a serious bursitis, active arthritis in right ankle joints, right thumb and indicator finger, left wrist and crippled four fingers, right shoulder and shoulder blade and also some pain in adjoining ribs.

On the 13th December I started with (the mussel extract). The first eight days, no change. On the ninth day increasing pain in all affected joints with slight fever till the thirteenth day (without fever and decreasing pain). On the fourteenth day all other joints which were affected in the preceding years showed symptoms of becoming active again accompanied by again slight fever. On the fifteenth day, however, I awoke for the first time with hardly any arthritic pain although stiffness and immobility still remained. From the sixteenth to the twentieth everything improved gradually, which caused a feeling of well-being. From the twenty-first to the twenty-third day another revival of arthritic pain and slight fever but now in all joints affected now and in former years. But on the twenty-fourth day this was all gone. From thereon a gradual decrease of muscle tensions, stiffness and a slowly increasing mobility in all affected joints. Swollen right knee and ankle slowly diminishing. On the thirty-second day able to walk again. On the forty-second day mobility, apart from some trouble of joint deformations, nearly normal for my age, hardly any pain, pleasant mobility! I am able to use all affected joints again without pain and with only some slight limitations and I can now carry out again the usual odd jobs around the house. I can walk again without trouble although I have to be careful with the use of my right leg as both knee and ankle joint were rather badly damaged.

Six weeks ago I had to pass my days, as a still dynamic person, in bed or on a couch. A sad prospect! Incidentally I also noticed a beneficial side-effect. Small cuts and skin grazes are now healing as I estimate, about twice as quickly as before.

P.S. My wife and I are sailing on the 10th of next month from Las Palmas on a world cruise which we desperately nearly had to cancel!

Although these two quoted excerpts are rather long it was thought appropriate to include them because they confirm several of the points made earlier in the book. They do also suggest that people suffering as seriously as this are quite able to give an accurate account of changes in their condition and are not likely to be easily influenced by quack remedies.

Fortunately not all cases are as severe as the two just mentioned. However, everything being relative, those people suffering other forms of the disease, can be just as desperate. The desperation felt by arthritics needs to be witnessed to be appreciated. Some of this comes through in the excerpts from the letters quoted below.

A letter from a lady in Italy indicates the joy and relief that come from simply being able to lead a normal life without constant pain.

I begin to feel like an agent in Rome as so many people have remarked on my wonderful improvement and want to try (the mussel extract) themselves that I am constantly getting it for someone.

You will be pleased to hear that I count myself one of the very lucky ones — not only am I restored to mobility, I am free of a constant pain that was really almost intolerable. I was taking painkilling drugs three times per day to alleviate the distress but since I finished my first course of (the mussel extract) I have not needed to take them. I have been able to get into and out of a chair without help, and have even tried knitting again.

I took a second course, following on the first bottle and now need the courage to stop taking them for a time to judge the long-term effects. The results for me are incredible and almost unbelievable. The best part is that I do not need any drugs whatever now. I have really gone quite mad and am doing all sorts of things which have been impossible for some time. Though I have to admit to being tired and full of aches I still do not have that terrible pain. There is a huge difference in aches and real pain. I only hope that other people will benefit as I have done. I am truly grateful and tell anyone who wants to listen to me just what happened.

The sentiments at the end of this letter and the desire for other people to benefit come out in almost every communication received. Obviously not everyone will benefit from this one type of treatment, but the sentiments in so many of these communications have been very influential in getting this book written.

An excerpt from a very short letter is an example of how the information about new treatments spreads around the world, particularly if they are effective. It is also an example of the fact that arthritic diseases are not restricted to the cold climate but are just as prevalent in tropical regions. The letter is from Nigeria where the mussel extract product is not yet available in shops. Obviously the writer has either bought the product overseas or had it sent by friends or relatives in another country.

You may be interested to learn that after one course my wife, who has suffered from arthritis for years, is now without pain in her joints, can bend and stretch much more easily and can now clench her hands — all without pain and without any side-effects. Marvellous!

As an example of the experiences related by people who have, or have had, severe hip problems the excerpts below are quoted from a letter received from a British seaman resident in London.

> I would like you to convey my sincere thanks to the staff that produce and market (the mussel extract). If the staff realized how much pain the capsules prevented me having in the last few years they would be very proud of what they produce as once again I say thank you one and all.
>
> My first benefit from (the mussel extract) was an increase in my sleeping hours. Prior to taking them I was fortunate to get two hours sleep in a night. At the present time I can get six to eight hours sleep free from pain. If anyone mentions arthritis to me my first words to them are to go on a course of (the mussel extract). I will keep recommending your product because I would like to see others get the benefit as much as I have done from the capsules.

It is not difficult to see how quickly the information about a product can spread when reading such letters. A letter received back in 1976 from a sheep-farmer's wife in New Zealand says:

> I would like you to know that (the mussel extract) capsules are helping my husband who has ankylosing spondylitis of the neck, spine and hips (for over twenty years). He finds considerable relief in his back and is able to drench sheep in comfort. He is fifty-five and his stoop had been getting progressively worse over the years. I thought I would let you know of his benefit as you are in a position to advise others.

The serious condition which this farmer is suffering cannot have been 'cured' by the mussel extract capsules nor any other medication for that matter. However, he is able to do his work without pain which to him (and his wife) must be a blessing.

Some correspondence received has advised of results that are difficult to credit to the product. It would not seem possible for a product of this nature to have such an effect. In fact it may be that it does not and the results were quite coincidental. However, similar reports have been received from several sources and it is therefore well worth reporting the stated facts.

In 1981 a lady in New Zealand wrote to advise that the product had allowed her to regain the use of her hands for routine housework, gardening, etc. She goes on to say:

> My joints are ugly and deformed, but still usable and able to carry on next day, even after hard work on the previous one.
>
> My new discovery is that, when restless in the early part of the night because of soreness and swelling and blotchiness in my fingers, if I take another capsule any time between midnight and 3 a.m. I am able within minutes to drop into a peaceful sleep and am unaware of the pain in my hands which look quite clear of blotches and slender when next I see them. They are white and active and ready to use in the morning. A most thrilling discovery and one I tell my friends about.

Another lady wrote from Australia to tell of the change in her hands.

> Going on a holiday trip to your lovely country New Zealand, I and my husband happened to have on our journey back home a fellow New Zealand lass. She noticed my hands and commented on them and then showed us a picture of her hands when she too had arthritis and had me sold on your (mussel extract) capsules. Well, cutting it all short I got onto them quick smart as anyone would give it a try. Well after my seventh bottle I began to lose the arthritis in ups and downs and my last bout was a real sizzler. But a wonderful thing happened. It was as if you got a cloth and wiped it all away, and that was two months ago now. Now tell me, can I reduce the dosage or keep the five a day still? I have put so many on them and they can see the results themselves. I had to give up bowls and gardening, etc., and believe you me I am so grateful to that young lass out from Queenstown who told me about them.

Whilst writing this chapter a letter came in from Christchurch

New Zealand which dealt with another aspect of the disease that the author would not have thought it possible to influence with the mussel extract product. However, the fact that the symptoms recurred when the lady ceased taking the product and disappeared again when she restarted does suggest that the condition was responding to the product.

> I thought I would put pen to paper and let you know that I have been taking (the mussel extract) now for approximately nine years. At first I started taking it for my arthritis which was at that time affecting my hips and found complete relief. However I also have had dermatitis or excema very bad since birth and many years had to be wrapped in bandages. As I grew older my skin always looked red and chapped so on taking (the mussel extract) I found my skin became not so bad or dry looking. I found this out after taking two bottles and then, not having any arthritis pain, stopped taking the capsules and after about a month my skin became red and itchy again. So now although I still get arthritis at times in various parts I take it all the time mainly for my skin. I thought I would write and tell you. It might help someone else.

There is a tendency to imagine that medical problems only affect the doctor's patients and never the doctors themselves. Of course this is not true and the author has several examples of people in the medical profession who have tried the mussel extract (mainly because of the freedom from adverse side-effects) with success.

In one case the person was a surgeon specializing in plastic surgery who was having to give up his profession due to arthritis in his hands. He used the mussel extract capsules and was able to resume operating.

Dr Christian Barnard, the famous heart transplant surgeon had to give up his work due to arthritis. After using the mussel extract capsules he too is back in the operating theatre.

Both of the above cases were verbally notified and thus direct quotations from correspondence are not available. They are quite genuine cases, however. In the form of a letter is the following report from a lady physician in Canada.

> I am over eighty years old and a physician with more than fifty years experience and can observe results with an objective judgement. My condition, spondylosis of the lumbal vertebrae, from which I have suffered for twenty years improved dramatically. I had tried many other treatments which did not help. My chronic rheumatism in both legs which made walking painful and slow, became so much better within only five days that I could walk again quite easily. I could hardly believe the result. After finishing the two bottles I tried to get them again but was only able to obtain a variety which contained an addition of Brewers Yeast, was darkish yellow and smelled of smoked fish. The improvement I had experienced gradually disappeared and the new capsules did not help at all.

The letter goes on to request more of the genuine product and indicates the danger of imitation brands trying to take advantage of a situation. Fortunately the product is now available in Canada.

Another example of people in the medical profession being willing to use the mussel extract for their own treatment is to be found in the excerpt from a letter from a State Registered Nurse which is quoted below.

> I am writing in praise of your product (the mussel extract). Nearly two years ago I developed rheumatoid arthritis of both wrists and spondylosis of the cervical spine. My doctor prescribed the usual anti-inflammatory drugs, but as a State Registered Nurse, and having seen the side-effects of these drugs on patients I have nursed, I was naturally very reluctant to take the medication.
>
> Leading a very busy life as a wife, mother and holding down a full time nursing job I decided to try other things. I tried homoeopathy, which turned out to be very expensive, and for me, not all that successful. Then I read an article about (the mussel extract). I toyed with the idea of trying it then at the company where I work as the Occupational Health Nursing Sister, I talked to a young man who is a sufferer of poly-arthritis (and has had

a hip replacement operation). He told me that he had a book about the green-lipped mussel which he let me read. I was impressed and decided to try a course of the capsules. This was in April this year. The book said that some people had to take the capsules for several months before experiencing relief. I was prepared to persevere. I was pretty desperate at the time.

I was very unwell, low in health and spirit. Unable to sleep at night, loss of power in my arms, shoulders, wrists and hands. I considered I was in the prime of life (forty-nine) and had got ten years or so to go before retiring from my nursing job. I found that in the mornings I could hardly lift my arms to dress and comb my hair. The pain was excruciating but I would not be beaten and continued to go to work each day.

I took the maximum dose of (the mussel extract) daily. Very slowly I began to notice an improvement by the summer May/June. The heat and swelling began to ease in the wrists. Then some days the pain would return to its maximum, especially if I was overtired or had done certain household jobs but somehow I felt I could cope a little better.

By the time September arrived, I knew that I was at last getting true results. Restful nights, a feeling of well-being, only the very occasional and mild ache in the neck, wrists, shoulders and muscles. In fact so slight to what I had been having that I could almost ignore the discomfort. Had I attempted to type a letter like this a few weeks ago I would have been in tremendous pain! I noticed that in October's issue of my magazine *Nursing Mirror* that someone had written to the 'Your Questions Answered' page stating that she and her husband had been taking (the mussel extract) for over a year and found them most beneficial. In fact it seems their results are very similar to my own.

This excerpt has been included because it is probably one of the best descriptions of the emotional and relief stages that sufferers of arthritis go through. The lady does finish her letter by saying that she is now taking two mussel extract capsules per day and that this seems to keep her comfortable.

The problems or worries associated with some drug therapy used in the treatment of arthritis are frequently recorded as the reason for people being so anxious to try alternative therapies. A letter from the mother of a girl suffering rheumatoid arthritis is an example of this. The letter is from Queensland in Australia.

> I am writing to let you know how well my daughter is since taking (the mussel extract). She has rheumatoid arthritis and she can use both hands now for writing and even raise them above her head.
>
> She only has 9 aspirins, 2 Brufen and 1 vitamin a day now and 1 gold injection a week compared with 12 aspirin, 6 brufen, 4 Codeine, 3 vitamins, 3 calcium and 2 Fergen. Before (the mussel extract) plus gold she has had three bottles of (the mussel extract) and now her hands look normal again, her gums do not bleed and her eyes are not sore all the time. She is still thin but she is eating well.
>
> One doctor we saw said he would not believe she had arthritis to look at her — if he had not read her chart he wouldn't believe it, he even took the name of (the mussel extract) to see if they could help others.

Another brief excerpt from a letter from a New Zealand lady says.

> Just a note to tell you how pleased I am with my husband's progress since taking your (mussel extract). He is sixty-seven years of age and has been a chronic sufferer of arthritis and rheumatism all his life, sometimes has been unable to move. After being in three different hospitals last year and taking so many drugs he became worse with too many side-effects thus upsetting a stomach ulcer. However, he has now taken six bottles of (the mussel extract) and the difference is really marvellous, moving around and able to tackle jobs around the house plus eating well and feeling much stronger.

It is always very pleasing to read that the patient has had the interest and approval of the doctor when trying the mussel extract product.

Fortunately this is now becoming a common situation whereas, in the early days, there was, understandably, a considerable amount of scepticism and reluctance on the part of the doctors to approve the use of such a strange-sounding substance.

An example of this patient/doctor relationship comes in the following excerpt from a letter from a lady in Auckland, New Zealand.

Some years ago I developed pain and stiffness in my right shoulder which was diagnosed as being due to rheumatoid arthritis. The doctor I consulted prescribed Brufen tablets and subsequently sent me to hospital where I underwent treatment, finally having Cortisone injections (which I might say were cruelly painful and did not seem to give lasting relief).

At times the pain reduced me to tears and I am not a weak woman. My only other relief was to sit in the hot pools at Waiwera where the thermal water gave temporary comfort.

I obtained a supply of (the mussel extract) pills and before taking them I asked my doctor if he had any objection to me trying the mussel extract. He said that he had no objection and would be interested to hear of my reaction to them. At the time they were not available as a prescription medicine, he said, but I was more than willing to pay for them and commenced the first course the next day. I did not experience any side-effects although I did notice some soreness in the first few weeks as described in your leaflet.

I am delighted to explain that I have now regained complete use of my right arm. I am able to reach up to cupboards over my head and to carry shopping bags, clean windows and perform most household duties. I might add that at the worst of my 'illness' I was unable to hold a pen firmly in my hand and was in almost constant pain — especially during damp or cold weather.

P.S. Dr ____ is delighted with the results of the treatment.

In Chapter 3 of this book reference is made to the feeling of vitality or well-being that almost all who use the mussel extract feel.

A letter from a lady in Cape Town, South Africa expresses this.

> In August last year you supplied me with two bottles of seventy-five capsules each of your product (the mussel extract) which I have since taken with extremely good results. Not only have the arthritic irritations in my elbows and finger joints receded considerably but I feel generally much fresher and more active than I did before.

Another letter from an Australian lady explains the good results she has experienced and concludes with the postcript.

> Whilst taking (the mussel extract) I feel full of energy and don't have that lassitude associated with arthritis.

It is important that people trying the mussel extract product realize that there may be a temporary increase in pain which can in some cases be quite severe. A letter from a lady in New Zealand describes her reaction.

> About seven years ago I heard of (the mussel extract) and discussed it with my doctor who stated that it could do no harm and if I wanted to waste money to try it. I immediately asked the chemist to send for some and started the course. Immediately the joints became even more painful and I could easily have thrown the tablets away but for my husband's powers of persuasion. Then, within about two months, I found I could walk short distances and was much more active. Six months later I took another course of treatment with still further improvement and decided to stop the butazone altogether. Since then I take a course of (the mussel extract) about every nine months and though I still have aches and pains while taking the capsules find that after each course there is still more improvement in the things I can do.

Finally, as far as the human aspect of the treatment goes it is worth explaining that a group of pensioners living in Florida, USA decided to carry out their own trial using the mussel extract. They documented all the results and were so pleased with the success that they asked a newspaper to give their trial some publicity in order that they might persuade the Food and Drug Administration to allow the product to be made available in the USA.

Unfortunately, despite their satisfactory results, they were not successful in persuading the authorities that the product was of value to American people suffering from arthritis. What is even more surprising is that a spokeswoman for the local Arthritis Foundation, which it would be thought had the interests of arthritics in mind, suggested that the results would simply be due to the natural remissive nature of the disease!

Thus, the USA is the only country where arthritics are not allowed access to the mussel extract product unless they get it themselves from another country. Just one letter from a lady in Georgia, USA is enough to show the feelings of the arthritics themselves.

Once again the F.D.A. has struck and we have been told that we can no longer buy the extract of the green-lipped mussel. For three years my husband, who is fifty-seven has taken these green tablets and has remained mobile. He even hikes up mountains, and bowls, not to mention tying his own shoes and navigating stairs. Before he learned of these he was on one medication after another, and each one had a side-effect that needed another chemical to take care of. The man was like a zombie and was time and time again in the emergency room for drug reaction.

Finally he threw them all down the john and searched for something else. A friend where he works told him about (the mussel extract). We found some and got the book to read. And read again. At this time he was not able to walk without a cane, could only navigate steps backwards and was unable to kneel, walk further than half a block or do anything — almost — alone.

After three months we began to see a change, and after that it was almost dramatic. He was mobile again and as long as he stays on (the mussel extract) he remains active and almost limber. His knees still swell and sometimes ache, but he is moving well.

Now it seems that the drug companies have pulled the rug out. We have a small supply in our fridge but what to do when that runs out? Can we buy direct from New Zealand? From Canada? Any other country? Please, what can we do so we do not lose out on these things? We do not want drugs again, we want these tablets.

If you will help us keep on top of these I will follow up any leads you can send us. Thank you for your help, we need it.

This letter is typical of so many requests that come from the USA. It has been included in full because it demonstrates the desperation of the people concerned to obtain something which they have found helps them and does not create adverse side-effects.

It is, of course, this very desperation which sustains the quackery that the authorities try to control. However, it is unfortunate that the controls are so sweeping as to allow only so-called 'proven drugs' to be available to people who have clearly found great benefit in another type of medication. It is also a pity that the arthritics themselves are not allowed to choose what best suits them and are not even supported in this by their own Arthritis Foundation.

Whilst this may sound rather emotive comment it is certainly justified when the cases of all those arthritics who died as a result of being given 'proven drugs' (which actually proved to be toxic) are considered. Surely there is an indication that the present system is far from satisfactory and could stand some revision.

Before completing this chapter it is appropriate to include a few excerpts from letters which relate to animals which have responded to the mussel extract treatment.

You sent me a bottle of (the mussel extract) three weeks ago for my fourteen-year-old cat about whom we were very worried because she was limping badly with arthritis.

The result of taking two tablets a day is almost unbelievable for she now gallops round our ⅓ acre garden. Yes it's true!

Also her coat is gleaming with health and she could, in my opinion, pass for a youthful four-year-old.

Labrador dogs are particularly prone to the onset of arthritic problems when they get old. A letter from Auckland, New Zealand says,

> I feel I must write you what is perhaps my last letter in praise of (the mussel extract). Chubby, our Labrador was put to sleep at Christmas and you may remember that she was one of the early animals to try (the mussel extract) some four or five years ago. At that time she had arthritis in the spine and hind legs and the vet was unable to do anything for her. From being unable to walk even the length of our driveway, once on (the mussel extract) she gradually progressed to become very agile, being able to leap up into the van, catch birds on the wing, etc. In fact she lived a normal, healthy and active life.
>
> Last Christmas she was frisky one second and paralysed the next — her spinal condition finally caught up with her.
>
> However, I am positive that (the mussel extract) gave her and us, five years of happy life which could not otherwise have been possible.

Another letter coming from England says,

> I have recently come within an ace of having to make the sad decision to have my beloved Labrador/cross bitch, Bess, put down owing to the progress made by her condition of ankylosing spondylitis. At only the eighth day after taking three (mussel extract) capsules a day she ceased to drag her right foot, ceased to walk (stagger rather) on the tops of her feet instead of the soles, due to loss of sensation, suffer less pain and began to regain interest in life. In a fortnight she was once again able to walk far more steadily and her legs stopped splaying outward.
>
> She has now recovered her ability to step up, over steps, where she had to be carried and is now going out for walks again, albeit walking slowly.
>
> She is thirteen (ninety-one by our age) so I think this is a remarkable result which I am sure will be progressive. Her coat has got a brand new gloss and I notice her eyes are fuller.

A New Zealand letter relates to a cocker spaniel.

> My cocker spaniel, is used for field-trialling and gamebird hunting in season and also rabbit and hare hunting so you can imagine he has quite an active life.
>
> Last January he started breaking down with very little work and limping around quite badly. My veterinarian X-rayed him and could not be sure what the problem was but thought that he might be slipping a disc in his back or suffering from a rheumatic condition. He suggested complete rest as a possible cure.
>
> Resting him did not work so I decided to try (the mussel extract) at the beginning of April. He improved almost immediately and has now had a very full gamebird hunting season over the last eight weeks without any signs of breaking down and in fact is working faster than ever before.

There are similar accounts to these which relate to poodles, alsatians and other types of dog.

To complete this section of the book two excerpts from letters describing the effect of a special mussel extract preparation on horses are related.

> The filly we are treating with (the mussel extract) has improved markedly after 3 months' treatment. She was X-rayed in December 1979 when the vet stated it was the worst case of arthritis and ring-bone he had seen that year. Butazolidine and Cortisone were given without effect — the filly's rump muscles wasted and some considered she should be destroyed as she became emaciated. (It was a back leg which was affected).
>
> As she was a throughbred filly and may have value as a brood mare, not to mention sentimental value, we started feeding her (the mussel extract). Now after three months she is fit, shining coat, well-covered, her back muscles have regenerated and she walks, trots and gallops with very little sign of a limp. She was X-rayed again last month and it was found that ankylosis had

taken place, the boney growths around the joint were smoothing and the joint generally had a tidier appearance.

The letter goes on to give more details regarding the filly and possibilities for her, etc. It finishes with the words, 'We are so pleased with her joint we are sending her to be broken in at the beginning of July.'

Finally a letter about a horse being used in pony club activities:

Maggie, an aged mare, developed serious lameness in December 1977 when the vet diagnosed arthritis in both forelegs. A treatment of Equipalezene commenced immediately with no dramatic improvement.

The treatment with (the mussel extract) was started on the 16th of February. Maggie did not find the smell particularly palatable but with persuasion and peppermint additive we overcame her objections. After the first week of treatment, the lameness improved and seemed only in the near fore. Her condition improved and she seemed more alert and was taking a lively interest in paddock activities.

Unfortunately, at the end of the second week she suffered a setback developing severe lameness of the off hind. A vet was called and Equipalezene given for relief of pain, the cause of which was undiagnosed. It was confirmed with the Veterinary Surgeon that the (mussel extract) be continued in conjunction with his treatment.

At the end of the third week, and completion of the (mussel extract) course, she was making a good recovery.

To summarize, Maggie has now a 'zest for life' that we wouldn't have thought possible three months ago, and apart from a weakness in her near fore, is in excellent condition.

These then are just a small sample of written communications, typical of those that continually arrive at either the author's office or that of McFarlane Laboratories NZ Ltd. Naturally there is also a considerable amount of verbal communication, even telephone calls from the USA, Canada and Europe.

The similarity in the reports is so striking that the author considers this type of information to be a valid indication of the effectiveness of the mussel extract product.

It is now left to the reader to decide whether the inclusion of such personal experiences as evidence of the value of the product is appropriate or is both scientifically invalid and indicative of quackery.

6
What the Future Holds

It has become increasingly obvious over the past few decades that significant changes in the exploitation of the world's natural resources are essential if these resources are to be maintained. Such changes have already taken place on land in that the efforts of the free-roaming hunters have given way to controlled farming of animals and food crops as population demands increased. Similar changes in the marine environment will see the expansion of aquaculture for both animal and plant resources.

In the field of medicine it is certain that research into the extraction and use of new therapeutic substances derived from marine resources will intensify. Already the properties of some algae and sponges have resulted in increased research efforts by those people responsible for seeking out new therapeutic treatments for the major drug companies.

Naturally much of the research effort will be directed towards those substances which may influence the course of the very serious disorders such as cancer and multiple sclerosis. However, there are also likely to be new additions to the available antibiotics, anticoagulants, cardio-vascular stimulators and anaesthetics resulting from current marine studies.

For medical research or farming of marine species to make satisfactory progress it is essential that pollution of the sea is controlled. Human nature being what it is, it usually takes a crisis of some sort to give realization to the fact that our natural assets are limited. When things are plentiful they seem to be taken for granted. Also, unfortunately, their rate of decline may not be noticed in time to prevent them being lost altogether.

Two factors which need care and attention result from earlier attitudes towards exploitation of and pollution of the seas. These are conservation of stocks and protection of the marine environment from polluting influences.

The preservation or conservation of stocks can be achieved by a balance between farming of the sea and regulatory control of non-farmed species. The condition of the marine environment and its inhabitants can be achieved by a much broader recognition of the influence of pollution.

Farming the Seas in the Future

It is reasonable to assume that current marine farming operations will continue and possibly enjoy refinements and improvements with developing technology.

Such farms will cultivate shellfish such as mussels and oysters, crustaceans such as prawns and shrimps, crayfish and lobster and various species of fish such as salmon, trout and catfish. This is by no means an exhaustive list of currently farmed species.

In the future it is probable that techniques will be developed for economic farming of certain seaweeds and more species of marine animals such as sponges or corals which are not to be used for food but for medicine.

There is little doubt that the technology for the cultivation of most marine species is already available but the means of carrying out such technology in an economically viable manner is not.

In some instances the cultivation of certain species of marine plants or animals may well be only to provide a standard and consistent stock of material for pharmacological research. In others, however, it will be to provide the source for valuable biomedical substances which cannot be synthesized.

The farms will be of both onshore and offshore types and will depend to a large degree on an adequate supply of clean, healthy sea water being available.

The Change in Medical Sciences

One obvious change will be the increased application of marine pharmacology in the treatment of medical disorders. This will apply in two ways. One will reflect the increasing use of new medications originating in the sea and the other will be the increasing use of marine organisms as models for the study of physiological reactions and stimuli.

It is possible that there will be a trend towards the use of cruder forms of medication rather than highly purified synthetic preparations. Whilst these preparations may be technically described as 'crude extracts' or 'unpurified substances' this terminology will relate only to the degree of chemical or biochemical refinement. It will not suggest a lowering of standards for hygiene, quality and safety of such materials.

The reasoning behind these observations is that it is recognized that crude substances (which contain the specific substance upon which our synthetic medication is based), can often be as effective as the pure substance alone without the disadvantage of adverse side-effects.

In most cases it can be argued that the only deterrent to just using natural crude preparations in the first place is directly linked to the difficulty of obtaining the large quantities that could in some cases be necessary and the inconvenience factor associated with using materials in this form. There are also instances where such crude preparations could be unstable and thus unusable unless freshly harvested.

It is considered, however, that some of the new discoveries in relation to medicines from the sea may need to be used in a crude extract form because extraction of the active principle or synthesis of it are impractical. Fortunately modern technology should allow the concentration and preparation of such medicinal substances in a safe, stable and convenient form for use. The mussel extract product is an example of this.

Changes in Pollution of the Seas

It is important when considering pollution of the marine environment, that the subject matter be kept in perspective. Pollution has become an emotive topic and is inclined to attract exaggerated statements. Unfortunately such statements sometimes do harm rather than good to the overall desire for a balanced, healthy environment.

It must be accepted that as long as animal forms (especially the human ones) live on earth, there will always be polluting materials created. The maximum effort therefore needs to be directed towards the most efficient disposal of absolute minimal amounts of waste materials.

Pollution is a relative factor. It is not always the most objectionable-looking or vile-smelling substances that are the most harmful. Some of the most hazardous and damaging pollutants are odourless and can have the appearance of drinking water.

It is well to appreciate that the muddy brown sea water flowing over estuarine and coastal beaches probably supports a far greater life mass than the clear blue tropical seas. In fact it can even be the dense concentrations of marine life which gives the water its turbid appearance.

Another point worth noting is that the influence of pollution depends upon several variable factors and not merely on the substance itself. For instance, pure clean drinking water is deadly to most marine species and clean unpolluted sea water is deadly to freshwater species. Thus a discharge of large volumes of clean fresh water to the sea is in effect polluting it.

Obviously the question of 'degree' comes into the picture and it is this factor which needs to be considered carefully when the future pollution of the seas is being assessed.

It can be argued that the addition of normal domestic sewage wastes to the sea is not harmful and may even be beneficial. Provided that the domestic sewage wastes do not contain detergents, insecticide or herbicide residues and such, then the statement is true. Sewage wastes rarely harm the marine life itself provided they are not at a level sufficient to deplete the oxygen content of the water. They may however, seriously affect the humans who consume the polluted marine species, particularly if pathogenic bacteria have been present in the sewage discharge.

Treatment of sewage wastes prior to discharge, whilst not entirely removing microbiological contaminants, significantly reduces the polluting effect of the residual waste. By removing solid matter the survival period for bacteria in sea water is considerably reduced and of course the numbers of bacteria actually discharged are also reduced. Aeration, removal of dissolved metal contaminants and other such treatments, if done efficiently, make the discharge of sewage effluent to the sea a relatively harmless activity.

Thus, although the idea of sewage going into the sea is unpleasant, provided these wastes are adequately treated and are discharged in suitable areas away from marine farms, bathing beaches or natural shellfish beds, they are unlikely to harm the marine environment.

Pollution by oil is a different matter altogether. In any form (although it should be remembered that crude oil is a 'natural' substance), oils are damaging to the inhabitants of the sea and seashore. Oil pollution almost entirely occurs as a result of human error. No amount of techonology will ever remove the human error element and therefore oil pollution will always be a potential problem.

The methods of dealing with oil pollution of the sea in the past have not been conducive to the preservation of marine life. These methods have been based on the principle that the most desirable action is to get the oil out of sight and prevent it landing on the beaches. Thus, emulsifying agents which allow the oil to form an emulsion which will disperse in water have been used both at sea and on the beaches. The result of using such agents, whilst beneficial from the point of view of bathing beaches and, of course, for seabirds, has been to increase the polluting influence for marine life in the sea and on the shore.

Crude oil (which tends to be the main type involved in accidental spillages at sea), is relatively non-toxic and biodegradable. If left alone it will rapidly change its composition. The lighter fractions begin to volatilize into the atmosphere, the remaining fraction becomes denser, attracts detritus and grit particles from the surrounding water and eventually loses buoyancy and sinks. On the sea-bed natural biodegradation of the residue will take place.

On the other hand, if the oil is emulsified, it then penetrates the whole water volume of the sea instead of just the surface. On shore, it is able to trickle into cracks and crevices, sink into sand and generally affect organisms which could otherwise have escaped its influence. In addition some of the detergents and emulsifying agents used can make the resulting mixture much more toxic than the original oil.

The message for the future is that oil pollution should be dealt with by complete physical removal wherever possible. Failing that, it should be left alone. Of course cost comes into the consideration of how best to treat oil spills, and physical removal could be the most expensive procedure. Fortunately methods for physically removing oil from the sea have been developed and in some cases, actually used. Hopefully these activities will lead to more design and development in this area to combat more of the future oil pollution in the least damaging way.

Pollution by radioactive wastes is a very sensitive and difficult issue to deal with. That radioactive wastes will continue to be produced has to be recognized as inevitable and therefore a disposal problem will continue to exist.

The present system of sealing radioactive wastes inside concrete-weighted drums which are then dumped in the ocean is not satisfactory. Evidence has already been reported of the leaking of activity from such sources, and the fact that powerful water movements in the deep oceans can transport even heavy materials like these drums to other regions makes the procedure unreliable.

At present there is little information available on the effects of radioactive materials on marine life. However, some forms of marine life have the ability to concentrate radioactive elements and, although they themselves may not be adversely affected, the humans who eat them may be. Certainly it would be undesirable for marine species from which therapeutic substances were to be extracted or prepared to be radioactive.

Whilst there is no reason to believe that such dangers exist at the present time, it is necessary to give consideration to the production of, and methods of disposal of such waste materials in the future so that the problem is never created. It is the type of problem that, once, created, cannot readily be rectified either by treatment or natural decomposition.

Possibly one of the least obvious yet most threatening and hazardous forms of pollution which can significantly influence the future use of the seas for medication and food supply purposes is that caused by pesticide and herbicidal composed residues. There are many forms of these compounds, probably the best known being DDT (dichloro-diphenyl-trichloro-ethane).

These chlorinated hydrocarbons are very resistant to biodegradation and take many years to break down into less harmful substances. The widespread use of pesticidal and herbicidal sprays has resulted in these substances being detected in animals as remotely situated as the Arctic regions. In the marine world they tend to concentrate in the fatty tissues of organisms and can pass right through the food chain from microscopic plankton to large mammals, being further concentrated on the way.

Whilst there is some controversy as to the effects of DDT and its breakdown products on marine creatures, it can be shown that this type of substance can adversely influence growth and reproductive functions. The results of such influences on the oceans' plankton production could have a serious effect on the human race irrespective of the direct influence on potentially useful marine products.

As these factors are already recognized then, hopefully, the future will see progress towards readily biodegradable and less hazardous products for pest and weed control.

The problems which have occurred in the past or could occur in the future as a result of the dispersal of industrial wastes are to some extent already being addressed. Unfortunately it took some unpleasant reactions in people who had eaten fish contaminated with metals such as mercury and lead to make some industries recognize the serious effects of untreated discharges of wastes containing these elements. However, there is now worldwide acceptance of the need to treat industrial wastes to a standard which will not harm the receiving waters, their inhabitants or those who feed on the inhabitants.

The gradual improvement, on the worldwide basis, in the technology of industrial waste treatment and disposal should ensure that this at least, is one area which will provide less cause for concern in the future.

There are two more types of pollution which are unfortunately still on the increase. One of these, thermal pollution, need not create problems if handled correctly.

Thermal pollution results from the discharge of very large volumes of heated water from nuclear power generating plants. Although the effects of such discharges at present are on a small scale when considered in global terms, they should be considered carefully in the design and expansion phases of future plants.

If used to advantage the discharge of heated waters, back to the environment from whence they came, can be beneficial. This could particularly apply in some marine farming applications. However, undesirable features such as the creation of imbalances in the local ecology through thermal differentiation of species and the creation of a thermocline (a sharp temperature difference between two horizontal layers of water caused by the heated water flowing over the top of the denser cold water), must be allowed for.

The other type of pollution is probably the least harmful yet the most obvious. This can be described under the heading 'flotsam and jetsam'. Since man first appeared on the earth pollution by flotsam and jetsam has occurred. However, in more recent times the nature of these materials has changed from simple, biodegradable timber to tins, glass bottles and finally plastics.

Apart from the danger to small boats where cooling water intakes can be blocked by plastic sheets or propellors fouled by floating synthetic ropes, the main hazard of these materials is the physical fouling of nets and structures used in farming or harvesting the sea. In addition such wastes are unsightly. This is, however, an area in which everyone can make a positive contribution. By practising decent habits and not throwing non-degradable rubbish into the rivers or seas it is possible for anyone to contribute towards the future cleanliness and aesthetic appeal of a resource which could well turn out to be the world's future medicine chest.

References

1. The Effect of Dried Mussel Extract on an Induced Polyarthritis in Rats, Cullen, J. C., Flint, M. A., Leider J., *New Zealand Medical Journal* 1975, 81, 260-261.
2. Pilot Study on the Effect of New Zealand Green-lipped Mussel on Rheumatoid Arthritis, Highton, J. C., and McArthur, A. W., *New Zealand Medical Journal* 1975, 81, 261-262.
3. Personal Communication from Kosuge, Professor T., Shizuoka, Japan.
4. Pharmacological Studies in Rat and Mouse, Roche, Japan, 1976, unpublished.
5. The Influence of Seatone (RO49-0282/100) and Fractions of Seatone on the Established Adjuvant Arthritis of the Rat, Daum, A., Roche, Switzerland 1976, unpublished.
6. *Perna canaliculus* in the Treatment of Arthritis: A Preliminary Study, Gibson, R. G., and Gibson, S. L.M., unpublished manuscript.
7. Gastro Protective and Anti-inflammatory Properties of Green-lipped Mussel (*Perna canaliculus*) Preparation, Rainsford, K. D., Whitehouse, M. W., Arzneim-Forsch/Drug res 30 (11), no. 12 (1980) 2128-31.
8. *Perna canaliculus* in the Treatment of Arthritis: Evaluation by Double-Blind Clinical Trial, Gibson, R. G., Gibson, S. L.M., Conway, V., Chappell, W., *Practitioner*, 1980, 224, 955-60.
9. The Anti-inflammatory Activity of *Perna canaliculus* (New Zealand Green-lipped Mussel), Miller, T. E., Ormrod, D., 1980, *New Zealand Medical Journal* 1980, 187-93.

10 Short Reports; Seatone is Ineffective in Rheumatoid Arthritis, Huskinson, E. C., Scot, J., and Bryans, R., *British Medical Journal*, 1981, 281, 1358.

11. Private Communication from Royal Melbourne Institute of Technology, 1980.

12. An Evaluation of the Toxicity of an Extract of *Perna canaliculus* (Seatone), 1. Acute and Sub-Acute Toxicity, Miller, T. E., Ormrod, D., unpublished.

13. An Analysis of the Teratogenic Potential of an Extract of *Perna canaliculus* (Seatone), Miller, T. E., Wu. H., unpublished.

14. An Experimental Investigation of the Pharmacology and Chemistry of Seatone, Couch, R.A.F., *Private Research Fellowship Publication*, 1981.

15. Anti-inflammatory Activity in Fractionated Extracts of the Green-lipped Mussel, Couch, R.A.F., Ormrod, D., Miller, T. E., Watkins, W. B., New Zealand Medical Journal 1982, 720, 803-6.

16. In *Vivo* Evidence for Prostaglandin Inhibitory Activity in New *Zealand Green-lipped Mussel Extract, Miller, T. E., Wu H.,* New *Zealand Medical Journal* 1984, 97, 355-7.

17. *Perna canaliculus* in the Treatment of Rheumatoid Arthritis, Caughey, D. E., Grigor, R. R., Caughey, E. B., Young, P., Gow, P. J., and Stewart, A. W., *Journal of Rheumatoidal Inflammation* 1983, 6, 197-200.

18. Seatone in Rheumatoid Arthritis: A Six Month Placebo-controlled Study, Larkin, J. G., Capell, H. A., and Sturrock, R. D., *Annals of Rheumatic Diseases*, 1985, 44, 199-201.

19. Six Month Term, Double-Blind Clinical Evaluations of the Effects of Seatone on Specific Arthritic Patients. Private Study at two Rheumatology Centres in France. Unpublished at time of writing.

20. Seatone in Arthritis, letter to B.M.J., 1981, 282, 1795.

Index